D1524476

# Color Atlas of COMPARATIVE VETERINARY HEMATOLOGY

## *Normal and abnormal blood cells in Mammals, Birds and Reptiles*

### C.M.HAWKEY, Ph.D. and T.B.DENNETT

The Veterinary Science Research Group and
the Photographic Unit
The Institute of Zoology
The Zoological Society of London

## *Section on Blood Parasites*

### M.A.PEIRCE, Ph.D., F.I.Biol.

Consultant Parasitologist and Corresponding Associate
International Reference Center for Avian Hematozoa

Iowa State University Press/Ames

Iowa State University Press
2121 S. State Ave
Ames, Iowa 50010

First published by Wolfe Medical Publications Ltd
2-16 Torrington Place, London WC1E 7LT, UK.
Printed by W.S. Cowell Ltd, Ipswich, UK.

First edition 1989

ISBN 0-8138-0449-3

# CONTENTS

# ACKNOWLEDGEMENTS

Most of the material illustrated in this Atlas was drawn from the archives of the Haematology Unit at the Zoological Society of London and we are grateful to the Society for permitting publication. Also to Mr D.G.Ashton, Mr O.Graham Jones, Miss Frances Gulland, the late Mr G.Henderson, the late Mr J.M. Hime, Mr D.M.Jones, Dr J.K.Kirkwood, Mr J.A.Knight, Mr R.A.Kock, Dr J.Lewis and Dr H.J.Samour for submitting blood samples to us and for providing the clinical background for the animals from which the illustrations are taken. Our understanding of avian and reptilian haematology was greatly extended by Dr H.J.Samour who obtained blood samples for us from many normal birds and reptiles during a sex determination programme which he undertook in a number of British zoos – we thank him and the Directors of Blackpool, Bristol, Chester, Edinburgh, Marwell and Paignton Zoos for their help. We have also received much interesting material from colleagues at The Institute of Zoology and from many veterinary practitioners and research scientists and we are grateful to Miss Mary Branker, Miss Frances Gulland, Miss Susie Jackson, Mr B.Allen, Mr A.Greenwood, Dr R.E.Purnell, Mr P.Scott, Dr F.Taffs, Dr J.Turton, Mr B.P.Viner and Dr A.Voller for their contributions. Particularly, we wish to record our appreciation of the collection of blood films from domestic mammals with haematological disorders, given to us by Dr Richard Evans, Department of Clinical Veterinary Medicine, University of Cambridge and of the slides of abnormal canine blood cells provided by Dr R.J.Slappendel of the Small Animal Clinic, Faculty of Veterinary Medicine, State University of Utrecht.

It will be clear to all who use this Atlas that its existence would not have been possible without the help and involvement of the laboratory staff who prepared the blood films and undertook the haematological examinations upon which it is based – we are especially grateful to Mr M.G.Hart, Miss J.Cowley, Miss M.Laulight and Mrs J.Henderson. Finally, we thank Mr D.Morris for his cheerful efficiency in unravelling several miles of computer print-out, typing the manuscript and compiling the species list.

# FOREWORD

Blood is a feature of all vertebrate animals and of many invertebrates. The significance of blood in humans and domesticated creatures has long been appreciated and featured in many ancient ceremonies and rituals. In the Old Testament (Deuteronomy 12, v.13) the writer describes blood as 'the life' and this illustrates its important symbolic role. Its physical features have not been overlooked, however; for many hundreds of years such criteria as colour and clotting time were used to assess the health of an animal or, in some cases, interpreted as important portents.

Despite historical interest, it is only during the past century that microscopical examination of the blood has become recognised as a valuable diagnostic tool. Haematology is now a well established and respected discipline within both the medical and veterinary professions but the body of knowledge which has been built up was confined, until recently, almost entirely to man and domesticated mammals.

Dr Christine Hawkey has done much to remedy this situation; in her twenty years at the Zoological Society of London she has built up a unique collection of material from a wide range of animals. The expertise she has developed has been put to good use; not only has it been applied to disease diagnosis and control in animals at the London Zoo but it has been made available freely to veterinary surgeons (and others) who have required information and guidance in the care of sick animals. She has always been most generous in her advice and many have benefited from her wise and good-natured counsel.

There has long been a need for an Atlas of comparative haematology such as this and Christine Hawkey was the obvious author – it is not only professionally and attractively compiled but is full of valuable information. It is truly 'comparative' in its approach since it covers mammals, birds and reptiles. Some will regret that amphibians and fish are not included but it is my hope that these will be featured in Christine's next book. The Atlas will prove of inestimable value to veterinary surgeons, zoologists, research workers and others who work with live animals since it describes both normal and abnormal features of many different species. An important bonus is that all the cases referred to were examined by veterinary surgeons so that haematological findings were backed by extensive clinical and/or *post mortem* data. An old French proverb states that *'Bon sang ne peut mentir'* ('good blood cannot lie'); in addition to descriptive morphology, Christine provides the technical information which will help to ensure that the sample is, indeed, 'good'.

Co-author is Mr Terry Dennett, who has been Head of Photography at the Institute of Zoology since 1973, prior to which he spent nearly twenty years working in the field of graphic art and photography. The high quality of the illustrations in this Atlas reflects his diligence and professionalism and will greatly enhance its practical value.

Dr Michael Peirce has contributed the section on blood parasites. It is paradoxical that, in many cases, these parasites have been the subject of investigation for rather longer than the blood itself; nevertheless, there are few good text books on their identification, especially in non-mammalian species. As one would expect from a protozoologist of international repute Dr Peirce's illustrations and descriptions are first class. He also has worked closely with the veterinary profession for some years and many of us are indebted to him for his help and advice.

I warmly welcome the appearance of this Atlas. Haematology plays a vital role in the diagnosis and investigation of disease and it is necessary to encourage its use routinely. In the past, such an approach has been hampered by the absence of a readily available and well illustrated text – there is no doubt that this Atlas will amply satisfy this need.

John E. Cooper, FRCVS
*Veterinary Conservator and Senior Lecturer*
*in Comparative Pathology,*
*Royal College of Surgeons of England*

# DEDICATION

To Gordon Henderson
Pathologist, The Veterinary Science Research Group
The Institute of Zoology
who lost his life in an accident in Glencoe on 22nd June, 1986.

# INTRODUCTION

Clinical haematology plays an important role in differential diagnosis and disease monitoring in man and is becoming increasingly important for the same purposes in other species. Examination of a stained blood film is an integral and, many would argue, the most helpful part of any routine haematological examination. In very small animals, where the amount of blood is limited, it may be the only procedure which can be undertaken. The ability to distinguish between normal and abnormal changes in blood cell morphology and to interpret these in terms of their pathological significance is one of the primary tasks of the haematologist.

For comparative haematologists this task is not easy, because of the large number of different species involved. For each of these an understanding is needed of the normal blood cell morphology and how it is influenced by different disease processes. Although similar principles are probably involved in all animals, in practical terms it can be extremely difficult to apply them when faced with the problem of assessing the blood picture revealed on a stained blood film from a less common species of mammal and even more so when the subject is a bird or reptile.

Clearly it is not possible to provide a complete picture of normal and abnormal blood cells of all species in one volume, even if this information were available. Human blood cells have been extensively illustrated and there are several existing books devoted to the blood and bone marrow cells of domesticated and laboratory animals, which concentrate mainly on presenting detailed information for individual species. The approach used in this Atlas is somewhat different. We believe that it is time to attempt a comparative survey of the subject. By doing this, it is possible to demonstrate some of the basic principles influencing the responses of blood cells to disease and thus to gain a general understanding of the subject. This eventually should create a situation where interpretation of blood films on sick individuals of *any* species can be undertaken from an informed background, whether or not the interpreter is familiar with the species in question.

All haematologists will realise that there are many potential pitfalls in this approach. Technical problems created by the difficulty of ensuring standardisation of staining reactions and techniques are inevitable, particularly as the materials and methods usually used are those developed for application to human blood and have rarely been modified to give optimum results on a broader scale. These variations can produce false indications of species similarities and differences. In fact, morphological variation does exist in the normal blood cells of different species, obviously so with regard to the red cells of mammals when compared with those of birds and reptiles and, perhaps less obviously so when considering white cell morphology, even among the mammals. Many of these differences are illustrated here, with the aim of providing some insight into the range of variation which can be considered normal. Inclusion of this normal material should also render the Atlas of interest to comparative physiologists, cell biologists and taxonomists.

Most of the material in the Atlas was drawn from the archives of the Haematology Unit at the Zoological Society of London. Extension of the scope into the realms of domesticated animal haematology has been possible by the inclusion of much valuable material from outside sources. The range of species from which the selection was made is relatively large, comprising about 300 mammals, 300 birds and 100 reptiles, but it must be borne in mind that the total number of species not yet available to us outnumbers this by several orders of magnitude. The normal blood cells illustrated are from animals in which good health was confirmed by veterinary examination at the time when the sample was collected. Although few of the animals were in a natural environment, there is as yet no evidence that blood cell morphology would be influenced by this fact.

The abnormal cells shown, in most instances, are from cases in which the diagnosis was indicated by clinical examination, response to treatment and, on some occasions, *post mortem* and histopathological follow-up. We have also included examples of cells which are clearly abnormal but where a definitive diagnosis was not made. This has been done to extend the recognition range of abnormal variation and, more importantly, with the hope of stimulating users of the Atlas to ponder upon the possible pathological significance of these cells.

Each cell or cell group is dealt with in a separate section. Each section is introduced by a description of the comparative morphology, relationships and function of the cells and comments upon possible primary and secondary pathological variations. Within each section, an attempt has been made to demonstrate the range of morphological variation considered to be normal in mammals, birds and reptiles, followed by examples of morphological variations associated with different disease processes. Each illustration is accompanied by descriptive notes and, when relevant, by details of cell counts and other haematological changes. As the purpose of the Atlas is to show how the blood cells of different species respond in a similar way to similar pathological stimuli, the illustrations of abnormal cells have been grouped according to diagnosis rather than to the phylogeny of the animal in which they were found. A species index is provided for those who prefer a less general approach.

Short sections on the methods used to prepare and photograph the films are presented in the Appendix. Animals are referred to by their common names throughout the text; a list of scientific names is given in the Species List. Unless otherwise noted, blood films were prepared from venous blood samples anticoagulated by mixture with ethylene diamine tetra-acetic acid (EDTA, sequestrene) and stained by the May Grünwald-Giemsa method. In most instances they were photographed at a magnification of ×100 or ×40.

# NORMAL BLOOD CELLS OF MAMMALS, BIRDS AND REPTILES

| CELL | MAMMALS | BIRDS | REPTILES |
|---|---|---|---|
| ERYTHROCYTES | Anucleate, biconcave disc (oval in Camelidae) | Nucleate, oval | Nucleate, oval |
| HAEMOSTATIC CELLS | Platelets | Thrombocytes | Thrombocytes |
| LEUCOCYTES: | | | |
|   GRANULOCYTES | Neutrophils<br>Eosinophils<br>Basophils | Heterophils<br>Eosinophils<br>Basophils | Heterophils<br>Eosinophils<br>Basophils |
|   MONONUCLEAR CELLS | Lymphocytes<br>Monocytes<br>— | Lymphocytes<br>Monocytes<br>— | Lymphocytes<br>Monocytes<br>Azurophils |

# Part 1
# Normal and Abnormal Red Cells

In all vertebrates except mammals, the red cells are ovaloid and nucleated. The red cells of birds appear elliptical in outline and have elliptical nuclei, whereas those of reptiles have more rounded ends and the nuclei are usually round. Mammalian red cells are anucleate and, with the exception of those from members of the Camelidae, take the form of biconcave discs. Camelidae (camels, llamas, vicunas, alpacas and guanacoes) have flat, elliptical, anucleate red cells. All of these morphological differences are strikingly obvious on stained blood films.

Also obvious is the high degree of size variation in the red cells of the main vertebrate groups. As a general rule, avian red cells are larger than those of mammals and reptilian cells are larger than those of birds. The largest red cells occur in amphibians, with the record held by *Amphiuma* in which the mean cell volume (MCV) is 13,860 fl.; the smallest are found in deer, sheep and goats. There is much interspecies variation, particularly in mammals where the mean cell diameter ranges from $1.5\mu m$ in the lesser Malay chevrotain to greater than $9.0\mu m$ in elephants, edentates and some large rodents. Because those animals with small red cells have high cell counts and vice versa, the normal packed cell volume (PCV, haematocrit) is relatively constant in mammals and birds. In mammals, there is some indication that red cell size is related to body size within a zoological family but this rule can be modified by environmental factors. Small red cells are found in species which normally live at high altitudes (e.g. some species of sheep and goats) where oxygen availability is low. These small cells provide an increased red cell surface area for enhanced oxygen uptake by diffusion. Diving mammals (seals and cetaceans), which are exposed to long periods without access to oxygen while submerged, have relatively thick red cells which act as a slow-release oxygen store. Apart from minor age-related differences, there are normally no significant intraspecies differences in cell size and, in most healthy individuals, red cell size is fairly uniform.

In mammals, birds and reptiles, erythropoiesis normally takes place in the bone marrow. In cases of anaemia and marrow dysfunction, however, it is not uncommon to find immature red cells in the circulating blood and, therefore, the recognition of normal and abnormal red cell precursors is of diagnostic importance. Little information is available on the process of red cell maturation in birds and even less for reptiles. On the assumption that, apart from differences related to loss of the cell nucleus in mammals, the process is essentially similar in all three groups, a simple classification scheme based on the developmental stages involved in mammalian erythropoiesis can be used to identify and compare immature red cells in the blood of other classes of vertebrates (Table 1). In mammals, the earliest recognisable cell of the red cell series is the proerythroblast which gives rise to a series of nucleated cells, the erythroblasts. These subsequently undergo the typical progressive changes associated with increasing maturity including reduction in size of both cytoplasm and nucleus, loss of nucleoli, decreasing cytoplasmic basophilia and assumption of functional characteristics. In the case of red cells, the latter involves the synthesis of haemoglobin and the acquisition of a shape suitable for effective gaseous exchange and for circulation through the vasculature. In mammals, it involves also the loss of the nucleus. The classification scheme derived from these observations (Table 1) inevitably is an oversimplification but provides a means of defining and, perhaps, of comparing the stage of immaturity of early red cells in the circulation of mammals birds and reptiles.

In normal circumstances, production of new red cells is equal to the destruction rate of outworn cells and this is determined by the red cell life span. There are marked species differences in the red cell life span which, in general, is directly related to metabolic rate and, therefore, to body weight. Thus, red cell survival is shorter and erythropoiesis more active in animals of a small size. There appears to be a direct relationship between normal red cell turnover rate and the rate at which an animal can replace red cells lost through haemorrhage or haemolysis; this is more rapid in small animals than in large ones. These points are important when considering indicators of active erythropoiesis which might be expected to show on a stained blood film or in a preparation stained supravitally for reticulocytes. In small mammals, it is normal to find a moderate number of polychromatic red cells in the blood film and the reticulocyte count relatively high. Such animals respond rapidly and dramatically to red cell loss. By contrast, in most large mammals, polychromatic red cells are rarely present under normal circumstances and the reticulocyte count is low. In some species, including horses and other Perissodactyla, red cells do not enter the circulation until fully mature and neither reticulocytes nor polychromatic red cells are seen in samples of peripheral blood, even during recovery from acute blood loss. In mammals, reticulocytes and polychromatocytes, particularly those produced in response to severe blood loss, are larger than mature red cells. The cells which enter the bloodstream under these circumstances are larger than normal in horses and other species in which circulating reticulocytes do not occur. In these species, a finding of macrocytosis is a useful indication of increased erythropoiesis.

In birds and reptiles, interpretation of samples stained for reticulocytes is somewhat of a problem

# Table 1

# A Simple Classification Scheme for Normal Erythropoiesis in Mammals, Birds and Reptiles

|  | *Mammals* |
|---|---|
| PROERYTHROBLAST | Large round cell, large central or excentric nucleus occupying most of cell. Nuclear chromatin finely stippled, nucleoli or nucleolar spaces present. Cytoplasm strongly basophilic. |
| BASOPHILIC ERYTHROBLAST | Smaller round cell, nuclear chromatin coarsely granular, no nucleoli. Cytoplasm basophilic. |
| POLYCHROMATIC ERYTHROBLAST | Smaller round cell, smaller nucleus in relation to cytoplasm, irregular clumping of chromatin. Cytoplasm grey or slightly eosinophilic. |
| ORTHOCHROMIC ERYTHROBLAST | Cytoplasm fully eosinophilic or with basophilic tinge. Nucleus reduced in size, uniformly basophilic or pyknotic. |
| RETICULOCYTE | Slightly smaller cell, no nucleus. Cytoplasm fully eosinophilic or with basophilic tinge. In Camelidae may be slightly oval. Reticulocyte stains reveal presence of one or more granules or strands. |
| MATURE ERYTHROCYTE | Smaller, fully eosinophilic round cell with central pallor indicating biconcavity. In Camelidae, fully eosinophilic, oval cell with no central pallor. |

because reticular material is present in virtually all of the red cells. In the earliest cells, this material forms a band of particles encircling the nucleus. During maturation, the particles are gradually reduced in number and become dispersed throughout the cytoplasm but some may persist throughout the lifespan of the cell. There are no firm data on the amount of reticulum present in the cells as they leave the marrow and it is likely that this will vary in different species. Several methods have been used for defining reticulocytes in birds and reptiles, including those cells which contain a complete perinuclear ring of reticular particles or those which contain five or more particles. At the present state of knowledge, evidence of active erythropoiesis in birds and reptiles is probably best based on the number of polychromatic cells present and on the appearance and size of the nucleus and cytoplasm in Romanowsky-stained blood films. Although systematic comparative studies have not yet been undertaken, there is subjective evidence that, as in mammals, small birds normally show greater erythropoietic activity than large ones.

### *Birds and Reptiles*

| | |
|---|---|
| PROERYTHROBLAST | Large round or amoeboid cell. Nuclear chromatin forming coarse open network with marked clumping. Large nucleolus. Copious basophilic cytoplasm with mitochondrial spaces. |
| BASOPHILIC ERYTHROBLAST | Smaller round cell, nuclear chromatin clumped, nucleolus smaller but still visible. Cytoplasm basophilic, no mitochondrial spaces. |
| EARLY POLYCHROMATIC ERYTHROBLAST | Smaller round cell, nucleus relatively small with clumped chromatin, no nucleolus. Cytoplasm grey or slightly eosinophilic. |
| LATE POLYCHROMATIC ERYTHROBLAST | Smaller round or slightly oval cell, round or slightly oval nucleus with irregular chromatin clumps. Cytoplasm grey to pale red. |
| ORTHOCHROMIC ERYTHROBLAST | Cytoplasm fully eosinophilic. Nucleus larger than that of mature cell, with irregular chromatin clumping. Reticulocyte stains reveal extensive cytoplasmic granules forming a perinuclear band. Granules become progressively reduced in number and dispersed through the cytoplasm. |
| MATURE ERYTHROCYTE | Oval cell, cytoplasm uniformly eosinophilic. Nucleus oval, elongated or, in reptiles, sometimes round. |

## Reversible changes in red cell shape

Apart from the basic differences in the shape of mammalian, avian and reptilian red cells and the variation shown by Camelidae red cells already described, reversible shape-changes occur normally in the cells of some non-human mammals which can alter the appearance of the cells on stained blood films. These shape changes are usually associated with the presence of haemoglobin variants which polymerise or crystallise under the conditions prevailing in blood samples being processed for testing and are probably correctly considered as *in vitro* phenomena. As yet, no pathological consequences of these phenomena have been described. The most striking is the sickling tendency seen in most species of deer and in some species of sheep, goats, antelopes and small carnivores (Table 2). In these animals, variants of adult haemoglobin occur which form insoluble, elongated polymers when in the oxygenated state. The presence of these polymers inside the cells leads to deformation of the cells into sickle, spindle, holly-leaf, triangular and other bizarre shapes, resembling those seen in human patients with sickle cell disease. The time taken for haemoglobin to polymerise in this way is longer than the length of time taken for the cells to pass through the arteries, providing one explanation for the fact that the shape changes do not occur *in vivo*. They are seen, however, in blood exposed for more than a few seconds to atmospheric oxygen as, for example, when a sample is manually or mechanically mixed or spread on a microscope slide during preparation of a film.

**Table 2**    Mammals in which non-pathological reversible red cell sickling has been recorded *in vitro*

| DEER | ANTELOPE | CARNIVORES |
|---|---|---|
| Indian muntjac | Nyala | Slender mongoose |
| Reeve's muntjac | Bongo | Blotched genet |
| Fallow deer | | Spotted genet |
| Persian deer | | |
| Axis deer | | |
| Hog deer | **SHEEP AND GOATS** | |
| Timor deer | | |
| Swamp deer | | |
| Sika deer | Domestic sheep | |
| Red deer | Soay sheep | |
| Père David's deer | Barbary sheep | |
| Mule deer | Mouflon | |
| White-tailed deer | Domestic goat | |
| Pudu | Markhor | |
| Roe deer | | |

A similar, less extensively studied shape-change phenomenon, associated with *in vitro* intracellular haemoglobin crystallisation, is seen in some other species of mammals. In these, the cells take the shape of the haemoglobin crystals. Examples of this phenomenon include the finding of square red cells in the mara, triangular red cells in the markhor and matchstick cells in the white rhinoceros and blackbuck. Haemoglobin crystallisation may also explain the occurrence of individual red cells which appear to break down into a number of small 'sickle cells' in the capybara.

## Inclusion bodies

Apart from intra-erythrocytic parasites, which are dealt with mainly in Part 5, Howell Jolly bodies, Heinz bodies or small, diffuse basophilic granules (basophilic stippling) are sometimes observed in the red cell cytoplasm. Of these, Howell Jolly bodies are indicative of diminished splenic function or abnormal nuclear division in man but occur with some frequency under normal conditions in carnivores, rodents, marsupials and small primates. They are single, eccentrically placed spherical structures containing DNA, which stain dark purple with Romanowsky stains. Basophilic stippling is manifest as the presence of a number of small, irregular granules, distributed throughout the cytoplasm and has been noted in mammals and birds. The granules consist of aggregated ribosomes and stain purple or blue with Romanowsky stains. Their presence is generally considered to be pathological and may be associated with lead poisoning or hypochromic anaemia. Basophilic stippling is sometimes seen in artiodactyls during the first few weeks of life, when replacement of foetal red cells by adult cells is in progress. In these circumstances it appears to be without pathological significance.

Heinz bodies are not seen in Romanowsky-stained films but, in samples stained supravitally with new methylene blue or methyl violet, they appear as one or more pale blue or violet structures of irregular size and shape, often associated with the cell membrane. They can be seen also in unfixed, unstained blood films as refractile structures within the red cells and under these circumstances have been termed erythrocyte refractile bodies (ER bodies). Heinz bodies consist of denatured haemoglobin and, in man, they are indicative of splenic dysfunction, toxic changes produced by oxidant drugs or chemicals, defects in the enzymes which protect haemoglobin from excessive oxidation or of the presence of unstable haemoglobin variants. In other mammals, their presence has been associated with phenothiazine treatment, brassica poisoning, onion poisoning (several domesticated species), maple leaf poisoning (horses), copper poisoning (sheep), exposure to methylene blue dye (cats), selenium deficiency (cattle), prolonged corticosteroid therapy (dogs) and 'wasting marmoset syndrome' (marmosets and tamarins). They have also been described in birds which have ingested oil from contaminated plumage. In some species, such as cats and common marmosets, Heinz bodies are not always associated with ill health and in others, for example the white rhinoceros, they can be produced artefactually during incubation of the red cells with new methylene blue. The haemoglobin of these animals may have a lowered stability threshold.

## Rouleaux formation

Rouleaux formation can be identified in the thicker regions of blood films and in wet preparations of whole blood where it appears as a face to face superimposition of the cells into stacks of various lengths and conformations. Rouleaux formation is confined to discoid red cells and does not occur in camelids, birds or reptiles. In man, in some other primates and in some carnivores and deer, a high degree of rouleaux formation is indicative of the presence of inflammatory disease. Among other mammals, the clinical interpretation of the presence or absence of rouleaux on a blood film is complicated by species differences; in horses and other Perissodactyla, for example, marked rouleaux is normal in healthy animals whereas, in most rodents and many Artiodactyla, it is rarely observed, even in individuals suffering from severe inflammation. The significance of red cell rouleaux depends, therefore, upon the species under consideration. Care must be taken to distinguish between rouleaux and agglutination. The latter is characterised by a close, irregular juxtaposition of red cells into clumps of various sizes, indicating an abnormal immune response, and is never seen under normal circumstances. In some species, the presence of intra-erythrocytic haemoglobin crystals can disrupt the spreading of a blood film in such a way that the red cells appear to be agglutinated.

## Artefacts

The biconcave discoid red cells of many species of mammals show a tendency for crenation in blood films prepared from samples collected into EDTA. This is considered to be an artefact arising from the general use of EDTA at a concentration which may not be isotonic with the cells of all species. Care is necessary to distinguish between crenated cells, which have no diagnostic significance, and burr cells or echinocytes, which indicate clinical abnormality. It has been noted that exposure to EDTA causes the red cells of some birds and reptiles to haemolyse. Affected species include crowned cranes, ostriches, kookaburras, tortoises and most species of Corvidae. Blood films from these animals should be prepared from non-anticoagulated blood or from heparinised samples. The presence of heparin imparts a blue tinge to blood films treated with Romanowsky stains and may cause clumping of the platelets and white cells.

In all animals, the breakdown of a small proportion of red cells is inevitable during film preparation and, whereas this is usually unnoticed when dealing with mammalian blood, the nuclei released when avian or reptilian red cells become disrupted remain visible and can cause confusion. They usually appear as amorphous, pale purple masses with an indistinct outline and are larger in size than the nuclei of intact red cells. Incorrect identification as lymphocytes or thrombocytes can be avoided on the strength of their lack of structure, indefinite outline and absence of cytoplasm.

## THE BLOOD FILM

Clearly, some background information about normal red cell size, shape and staining characteristics is required for the species in question in order to assess the possible pathological significance of these parameters in a given clinical case. In normal adult animals, the cells can be expected to appear as regular discs or elliptocytes, either nucleated or not according to the class of animals from which they come. Since the mean cell haemoglobin concentration (MCHC) is similar in all mammals and birds, mammalian and avian red cells normally should appear fully haemoglobinised. However, the significance of observations relating to the degree of polychromasia, the size of the cells and, in many instances, their shape, can depend upon the characteristics of the species under examination. For example, poikilocytosis is extremely common in blood samples from deer and other mammals with a non-pathological sickling tendency and in those with enhanced haemoglobin crystallisation but is rare in Camelidae under any circumstances. Overt macro- or microcytosis cannot be defined without knowledge of the normal MCV for the species. The possible significance of Howell Jolly bodies, Heinz bodies and rouleaux formation must be considered according to species. Care must be taken to distinguish between true burr cells (echinocytes) and the crenated cells produced artefactually in EDTA samples from many mammals. As a general rule, the morphological observations most consistently indicative of underlying pathology are hypochromia, spherocytes, target cells, agglutination, the presence in the blood of large numbers of immature cells and evidence of abnormal cell division. The significance and distribution of these and some other morphological variants are shown in Table **3**.

**Table 3**   Significance of some red cell morphological changes

| Observation | Indication | Mammals | Birds and Reptiles |
|---|---|---|---|
| HYPOCHROMIA | Anaemia, mineral (iron) deficiency | Significant | Significant |
| POIKILOCYTOSIS | Metabolic defect, increased erythropoiesis | Significant | Significant |
| ANISOCYTOSIS | Metabolic defect, increased erythropoiesis | Significant if no tendency for Hb polymerisation | Significant |
| TARGET CELLS (LEPTOCYTES) | Liver disease, hypochromic anaemia | Significant | Not described |
| STOMATOCYTES | Liver disease, haemolytic anaemia | Significant | Not described |
| SPHEROCYTES | Haemolytic anaemia | Significant | Not described |
| BURR CELLS (ECHINOCYTES) | Uraemia, hyperthyroidism, hypertonicity | Significant | Not described |
| SCHISTOCYTES | Disseminated intra-vascular coagulation, micro-angiopathic anaemia, severe sepsis etc. | Significant | Not described |
| HOWELL JOLLY BODIES | Hyposplenism, abnormal nuclear division | Significant in some species | Probably significant |
| BASOPHILIC STIPPLING | Iron deficiency, lead poisoning | Significant in adults | Significant |
| HEINZ BODIES | Exposure to oxidants, unstable Hb, enzyme defects, hyposplenism | Significant in some species | Significant |

**1-16** *Normal species variation in red cell size. The blood films were prepared from the blood of healthy adult animals and are printed at the same magnification. The normal range for mean cell volume (MCV) is given for each species illustrated.*

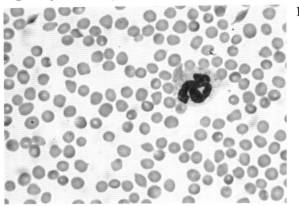

**1** Small red cells from a domestic goat (MCV 19-24 fl).

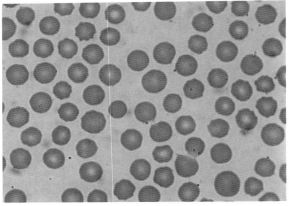

**2** Intermediate-sized red cells from a domestic cow (MCV 40-60 fl).

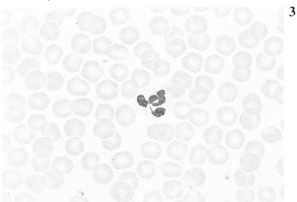

**3** Intermediate-sized red cells from a dog (MCV 70-85 fl).

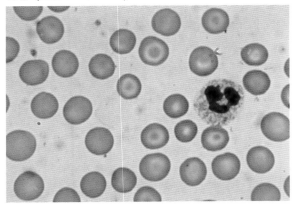

**4** Relatively large red cells from a Canadian beaver (MCV 92-110 fl).

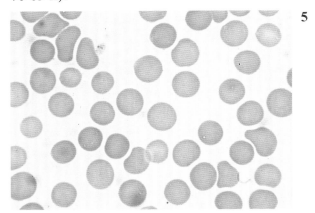

**5** Red cells from a bottle-nosed dolphin; they appear smaller than those of the Indian elephant, although their MCV is similar (MCV 100-120 fl) because, like the red cells of other diving mammals, they are thicker than those of terrestrial mammals and probably act as a slow release oxygen store during diving.

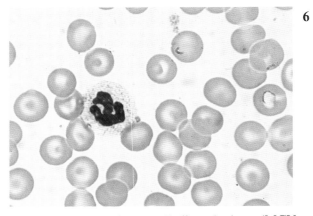

**6** Large red cells from an Indian elephant (MCV 112-130 fl). The red cells of elephants often appear as target cells on air-dried blood films. This is an artefact associated with their large size.

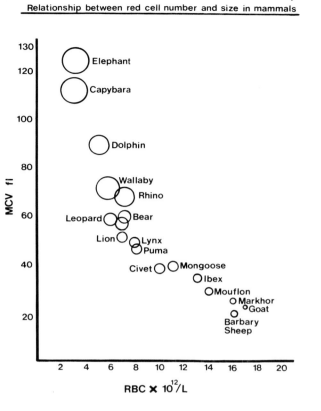

7 The relationship between red cell size and number. The cells are drawn according to their mean cell diameter. *N.B.* The position occupied by the bottle-nosed dolphin is consistent with an increased mean cell average thickness.

8 Comparison of red cell size and thickness in various mammals. The cells of the pilot whale are thicker than those of other non-diving species.

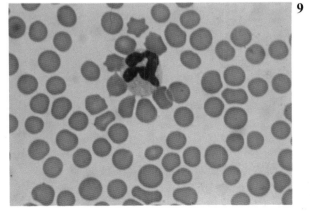

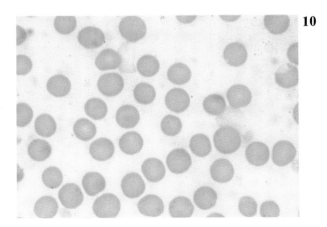

9 Red cells and a neutrophil from a healthy horse (MCV 40-56 fl). The neutrophil has agranular cytoplasm.

10 Red cells from a healthy donkey (MCV 57-70 fl). These cells are larger than those of horses.

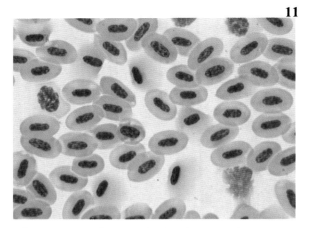

**11** Red cells from a budgerigar (MCV 99-105 fl).In general, avian red cells are large compared with those of most mammals; the size may be directly related to body size.

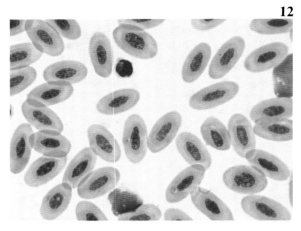

**12** Red cells from a common buzzard (MCV 150-170 fl).

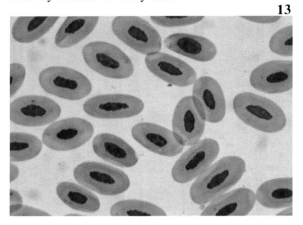

**13** Red cells from an emu (MCV 250-280 fl).

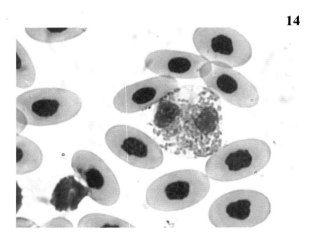

**14** Red cells from a common iguana (MCV 250-290 fl). Reptilian red cells are usually larger than those of birds. A normal heterophil is also shown.

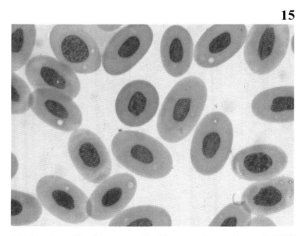

**15** Red cells from an Indian rock python (MCV 290-333 fl).

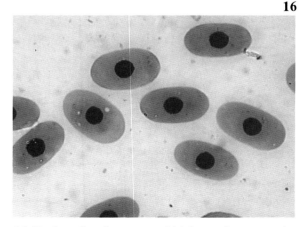

**16** Red cells from an Aldabra giant tortoise (MCV 400 fl).

**17-37** *Normal variation in red cell shape.*

**17** Scanning electron micrograph (SEM) of red cells from a healthy masked palm civet showing the bioconcave discoid shape common to most mammals.

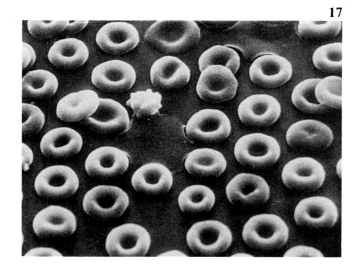
**17**

**18** Elliptical red cells from a bactrian camel. Elliptocytes occur in all members of the Camelidae. The outline of these cells always appears slightly indistinct on stained blood films.

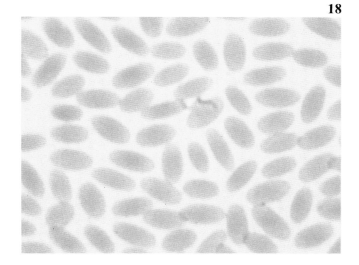
**18**

**19** SEM of alpaca elliptocytes showing the absence of a central depression.

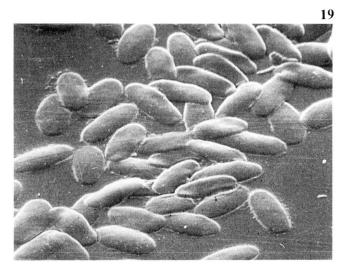
**19**

**20** SEM of North American turkey red cells, each with a nuclear bulge.

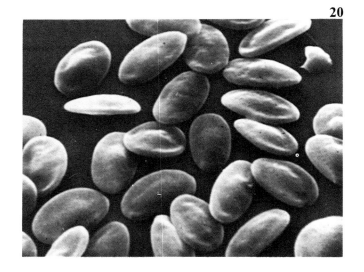

**21** SEM of red cells from a red-eared terrapin. Reptilian red cells are flatter and appear thinner than those of birds. No nuclear bulge is apparent.

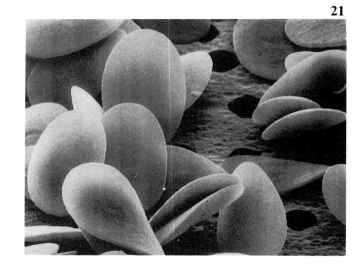

**22** Sickled red cells in an oxygenated blood sample from a healthy adult red deer (×40). Reversible sickling is shown by the red cells of adult individuals of most species of deer, some bovine and caprine animals and some small carnivores. In these animals, sickling is an *in vitro* phenomenon and is not associated with any abnormal clinical signs. The shape change occurs as a result of the presence of haemoglobin variants which form insoluble tactoids when oxygenated. Several different sickling haemoglobins have been described, all of which are different from human Hb-S.

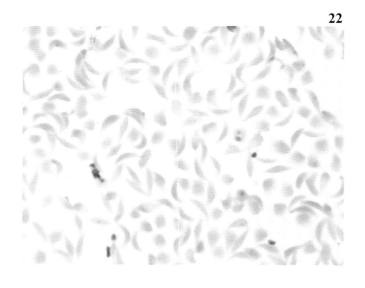

**23** Discocytic red cells and two neutrophils from a normal reindeer. Red cell sickling has not been found in this species.

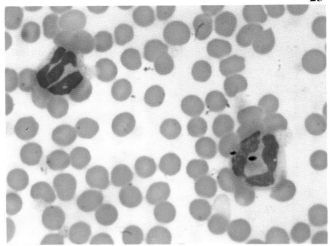

**24** Typical appearance of red cells in a fresh film prepared from venous blood of a 'sickling' species of deer, in this case an adult Père David's deer. Partial oxygenation of the sample during preparation of the film accounts for the presence of some sickled cells.

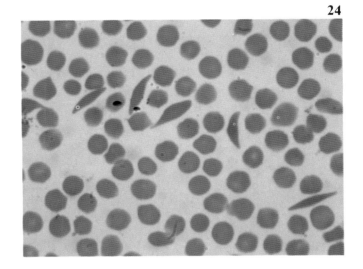

**25** SEM of sickled red cells in an oxygenated blood sample from a swamp deer. Many sickle cells, one spindle-shaped cell and several normal cells are present.

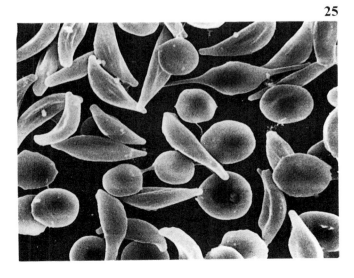

**26** SEM showing cell deformation in oxygenated blood from a Reeve's muntjac with a sickling haemoglobin variant. Sickle cells, echinocytes, spur cells and holly-leaf cells are present.

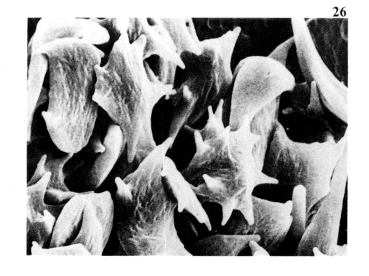

**27** Minimal red cell deformation in a fresh, unmixed, blood sample from a blotched genet (×40).

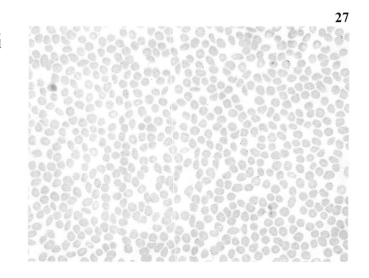

**28** All red cells sickled in the same sample as **27** after exposure to oxygen (×40).

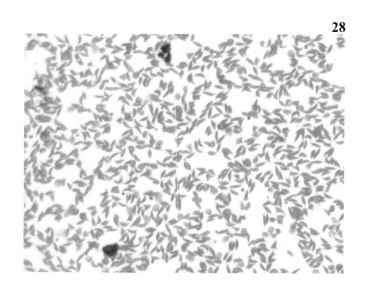

**29** 'Microsickles' from a capybara. Individual red cells appear to break up into several small sickle or diamond-shaped fragments.

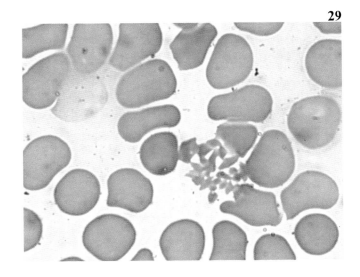

**30** 'Matchstick' cells, found in the blood of a healthy adult white rhinoceros. They are associated with the presence of a haemoglobin variant which crystallises in the same form. The film was stained supravitally with new methylene blue before the May-Grunwald-Geimsa technique was applied and a few of the cells contain Heinz bodies. This finding is common and without clinical significance.

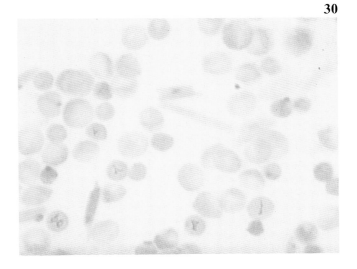

**31** Haemoglobin crystals from haemolysed blood of the rhinoceros in **30**.

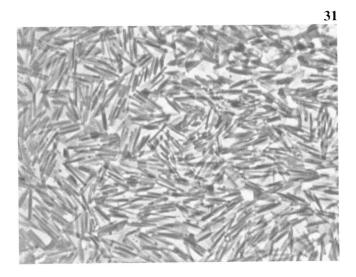

**32** Intracellular haemoglobin crystallisation in a capybara. Red cells containing crystals interfere with the spreading of the film and this can give the impression of autoagglutination.

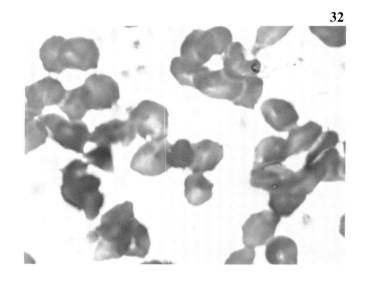

**33** Triangular red cells caused by intracellular haemoglobin crystallisation in a markhor. Adults of this species have extremely small red cells (MCV 15-19 fl).

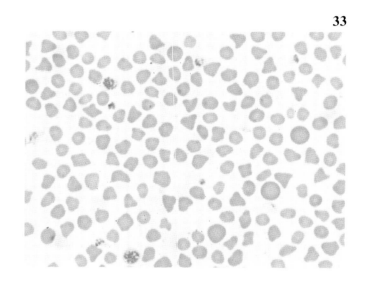

**34** Square and diamond-shaped red cells due to intracellular haemoglobin crystallisation in a mara.

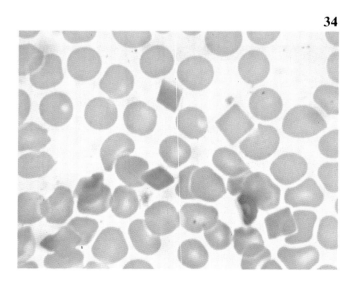

**35** Haemoglobin crystals in dog blood after prolonged storage in EDTA.

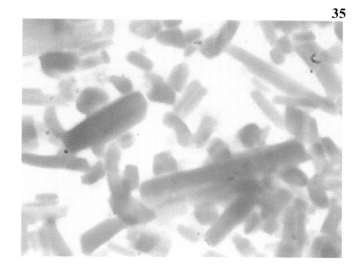

**36** Unusual red cell morphology in a hill mynah. This shape-change is reversible; its significance has not yet been determined.

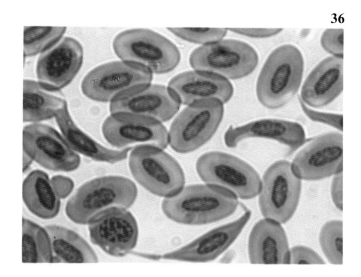

**37** Apparent intracellular haemoglobin crystallisation in a taipan snake.

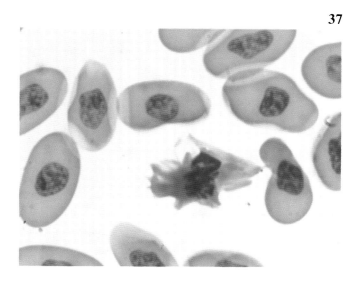

**38-54** *Miscellaneous variations in red cell morphology found in healthy animals.*

**38** Anisocytosis in a normal adult tiger. The red cells of most healthy mammals show a moderate amount of size variation.

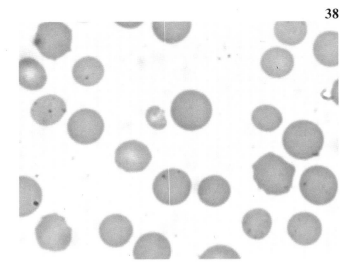
38

**39** Two red cells containing Howell Jolly bodies from a red-necked wallaby. These represent nuclear remnants and are often found in small numbers in healthy marsupials, feline animals, rodents and small primates.

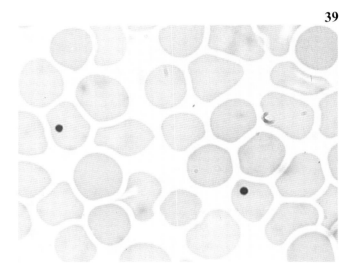
39

**40** Two red cells containing Howell Jolly bodies from a brown capuchin monkey.

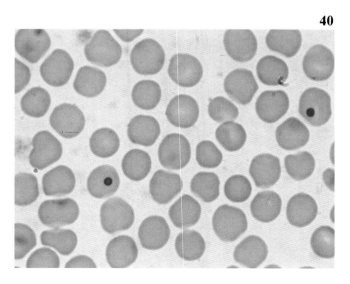
40

**41** Accentuated rouleaux formation in the blood of a healthy Przewalski's wild horse. This is a normal finding in equine animals, elephants and some other mammalian species. In these animals the erythrocyte sedimentation rate is always rapid and does not give a useful indication of clinical status. An eosinophil with the strikingly obvious cytoplasmic granules, typical of domestic and wild horses, is present.

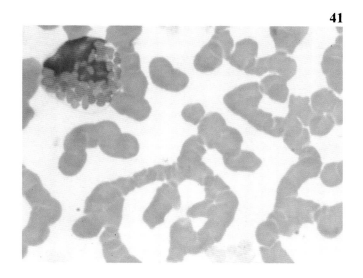

**42** Red cells containing Heinz bodies from a healthy cat (new methylene blue stain). It is relatively common to find these inclusions in feline red cells and, when present in small numbers, they are generally considered to be without clinical significance. Note the close association between Heinz bodies and cell membrane.

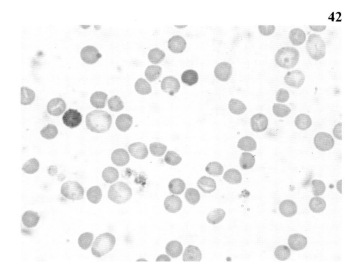

**43** Heinz bodies and a few reticulocytes in the blood of a healthy common marmoset (new methylene blue and rhodanile blue stain).

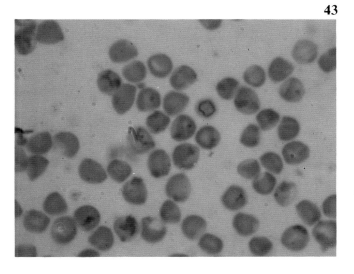

**44** A red cell containing a Cabot's ring in blood from a healthy llama (new methylene blue stain). These thread-like rings and convolutions are thought to be artefacts representing denatured membrane protein and are frequently found in the blood of normal Camelidae.

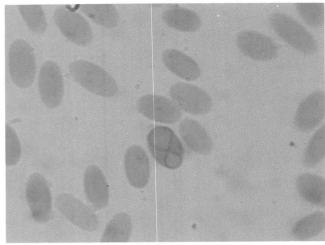

**45** An erythroplastid from a healthy budgerigar. The presence of a small number of anucleate red cells in the blood of birds and reptiles has no pathological significance. Three polychromatic erythroblasts are also present.

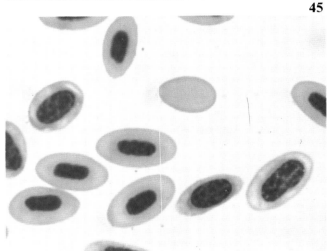

**46-49** *Examples of active erythropoiesis in small mammals and birds. The red cell survival time is short in small animals with a high basal metabolic rate and evidence of active erythropoiesis, such as the presence of polychromasia, circulating erythroblasts and, in mammals, a high reticulocyte count, is considered normal in these animals.*

**46** Polychromasia and a polychromatic erythroblast in a healthy adult mouse lemur. A normal lymphocyte with cytoplasm containing granules is also shown.

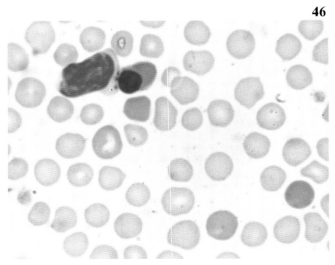

**47** Numerous reticulocytes in the blood of a healthy adult red-bellied tamarin (new methylene blue stain).

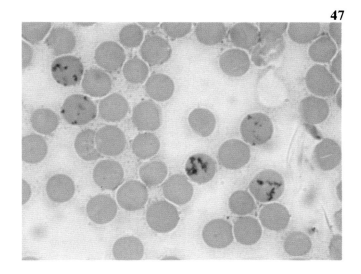

**48** Mature red cells, basophilic, polychromatic and orthochromic erythroblasts in the blood of a normal adult budgerigar. The nuclear size decreases and the amount of cytoplasm increases as the cells mature. Two of the basophilic erythroblasts have not yet become elliptical.

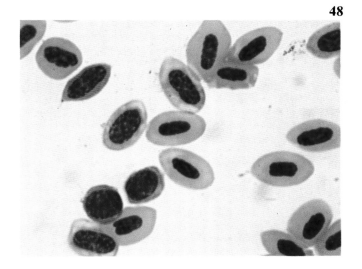

**49** A binucleated polychromatic erythroblast from the budgerigar in **48**.

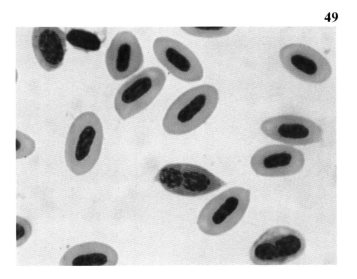

**50** Three basophilic erythroblasts in the blood of an immature cattle egret. Regenerative anaemia is often found in young birds and usually resolves without treatment.

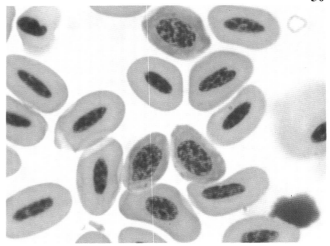

**51** Red cell precursors in a bone marrow sample from a healthy grey heron. All developmental stages from proerythroblast to mature red cells are present.

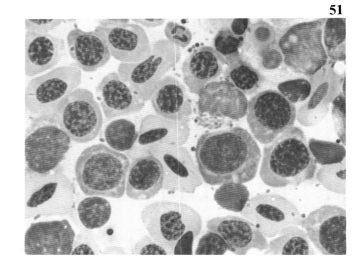

**52** Active erythropoiesis in a healthy brown python. Two polychromatic erythroblasts are illustrated, which appear microcytic compared with the mature cells. Cytoplasmic vacuolation is often seen in the erythroblasts of normal snakes.

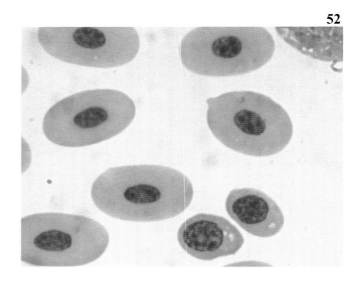

**53** A polychromatic erythroblast with vacuolated cytoplasm from a healthy Indian python.

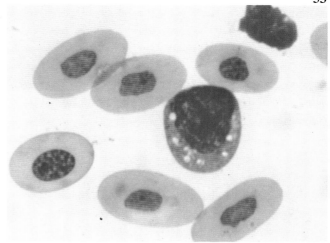

**54** Orthochromic erythroblasts and mature red cells from a healthy greater plated lizard.

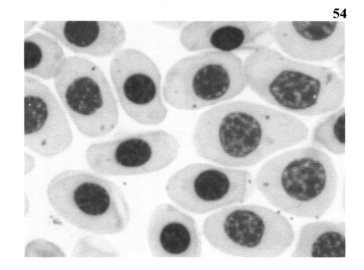

**55-63** *Common artefacts affecting red cells.*

**55** Crenated red cells in an EDTA sample from a normal guinea pig. Crenation is frequently seen in mammalian blood samples collected into commercially available EDTA tubes. Crenation of the elliptical cells of Camelidae, birds and reptiles does not occur.

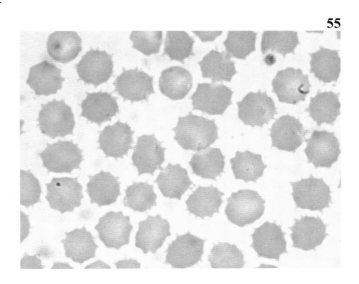

**56** Crenation and anisocytosis in an EDTA sample from a normal leopard.

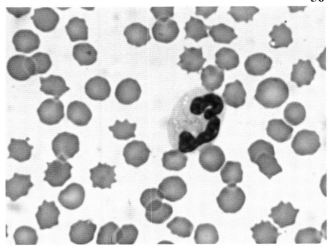

**57** Crenated red cells in an EDTA blood sample from a healthy domestic pig.

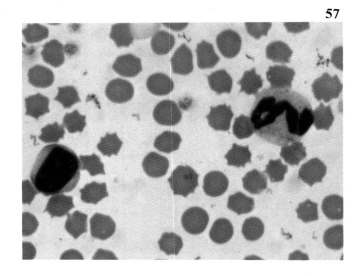

**58** Marked crenation in an EDTA sample from a normal ruffed lemur.

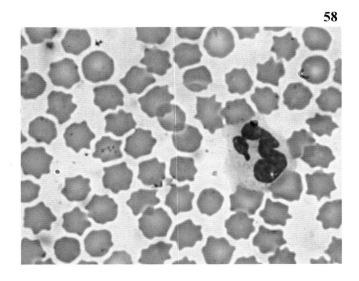

**59** Poorly fixed cockatoo red cells showing nuclear 'bleeding'.

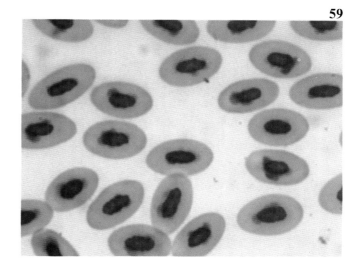

**60** Normal red cells and amorphous purple-staining material originating from the nuclei of disrupted red cells from a healthy wood pigeon (×40). Breakdown of a small number of red cells commonly occurs during the preparation of films from avian and, less often, from reptilian blood samples. Unless large numbers of cells are affected, this artefact can be disregarded. Care must be taken to avoid the misidentification of red cell nuclei as lymphocytes or thrombocytes.

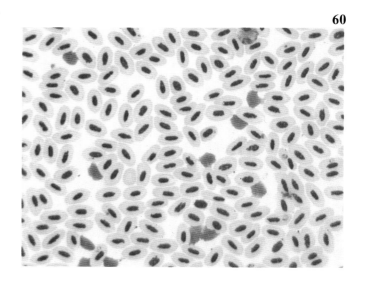

**61** Stages in red cell breakdown leading to the presence of amorphous nuclear material in a blood film from a normal spoonbill.

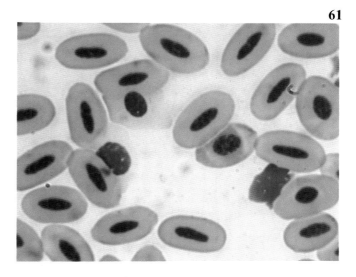

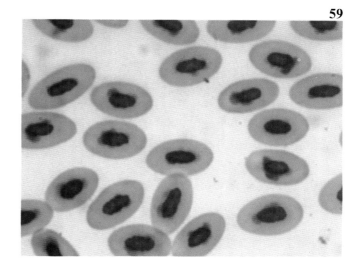

**62** Many haemolysed red cells in an EDTA sample from a crowned crane (×40). Blood samples from this species and from several other groups of birds and reptiles including ostriches, kookaburras, corvids and tortoises, undergo haemolysis when mixed with EDTA although not with heparin or citrate. The reason is not known.

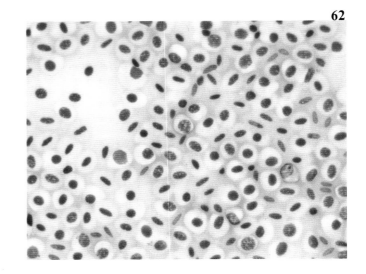

**63** Red cell lysis in an EDTA sample from an Aldabra giant tortoise.

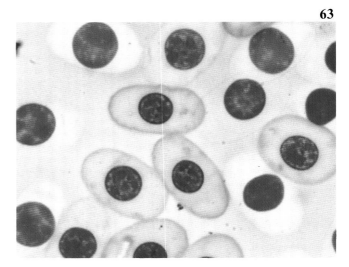

**64-150** *Abnormal variations in red cell morphology.*

**64** Iron deficiency anaemia in a dog. The red cells are hypochromic and slightly microcytic. Active erythropoiesis is indicated by the presence of polychromatic cells. The platelets show anisocytosis.

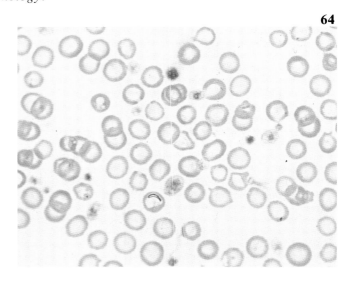

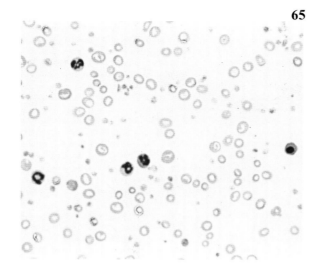

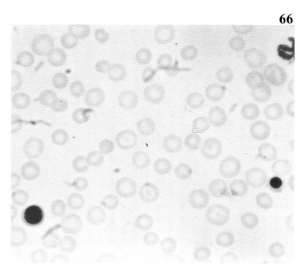

**65** Severe hypochromic anaemia in a cat with *Haemobartonella felis* parasites (×40). The red cells also show anisocytosis and one nucleated red cell (normoblast, orthochromic erythroblast) is present.

**66** Regenerative hypochromic anaemia in a dog. Target cells, two orthochromic erythroblasts and a normal neutrophil are present.

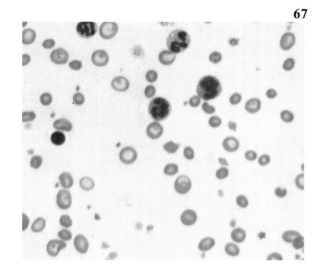

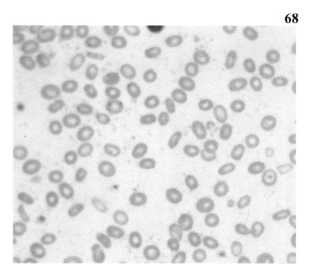

**67** Marked anisocytosis, neutrophilia and thrombocytosis in a dog with severe regenerative hypochromic anaemia associated with hormonal imbalance (×40, Hb 3.3 g/dl).

**68** Blood from the dog in **67**, showing the presence of elliptocytes during the recovery period (×40, Hb 8.1 g/dl).

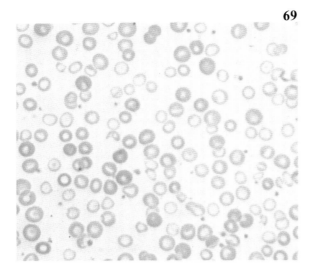

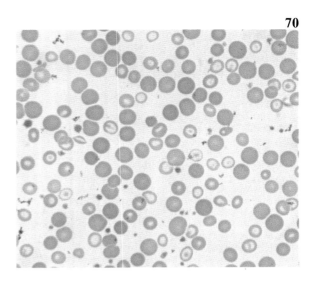

**69** Iron deficiency anaemia resulting from chronic blood loss in a lion-tailed macaque with menorrhagia (×40, Hb 4.0 g/dl). The red cells are hypochromic and microcytic.

**70** The macaque in **69**, 10 days after iron treatment (×40, Hb 7.2 g/dl). There is now a population of normochromic normocytic red cells.

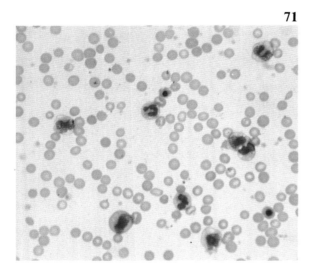

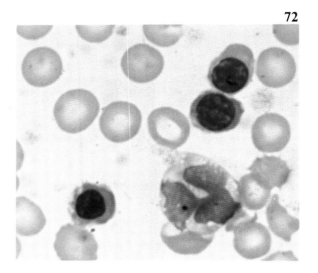

**71** Erythroblasts and leucocytosis in a silvery marmoset with regenerative haemorrhagic anaemia (×25, Hb 7.2 g/dl).

**72** A higher magnification of two polychromatic and one orthochromic erythroblasts from the marmoset in **71**. The red cells show hypochromia and polychromasia. An effete leucocyte is present.

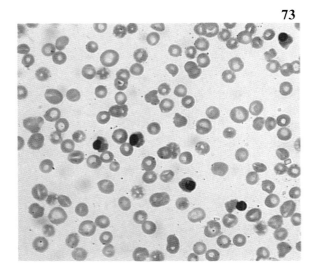

**73**

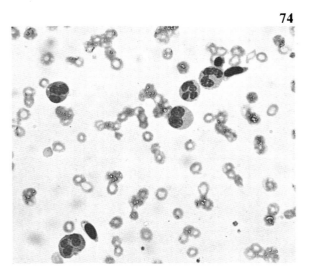

**74**

**73** Red cells showing anisocytosis, hypochromia, stomatocytosis and polychromasia from an owl monkey with regenerative anaemia (×40, Hb 5.3 g/dl). Many erythroblasts are present.

**74** Abnormal erythropoiesis in an owl monkey with severe regenerative hypochromic anaemia (×40). There are two misshapen and one normal erythroblasts in the field.

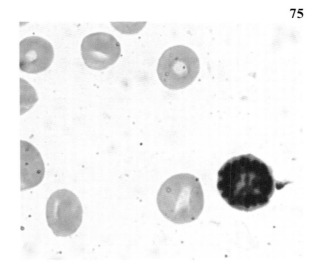

**75**

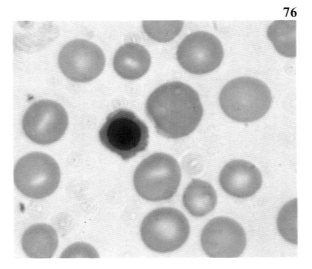

**76**

**75** A mitotic erythroblast from the owl monkey in **74**.

**76** Anisocytosis, polychromasia and a polychromatic erythroblast in a red bellied tamarin with regenerative haemorrhagic anaemia (Hb 5.3 g/dl).

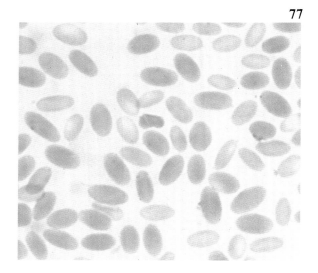

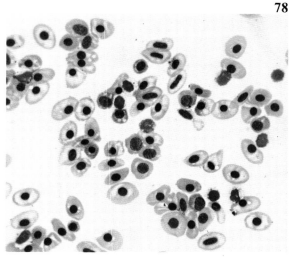

**77** Hypochromia and anisocytosis associated with copper deficiency in a bactrian camel.

**78** Severe hypochromic anaemia in a domestic duck (×40, Hb 3.4 g/dl, MCHC <20 g/dl). The cells show vacuolation, anisocytosis and shape variation and many have abnormally round, condensed nuclei. The presence of polychromatic erythroblasts indicates active erythropoiesis.

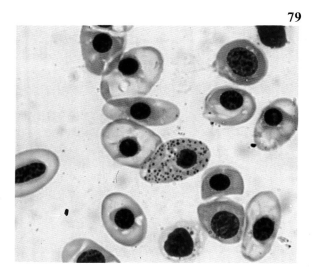

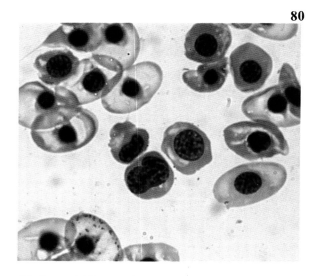

**79** A higher magnification of red cells from the duck in **78**. Hypochromia and active erythropoiesis is clearly evident and one cell shows basophilic stippling (punctate basophilia).

**80** Basophilic erythroblasts with abnormal nuclear division from the duck in **78**.

**81** Hypochromia, anisocytosis, microcytosis and poikilocytosis in a whooper swan with lead poisoning (Hb 5.9 g/dl). Two normal thrombocytes with vacuolated cytoplasm are present in the field.

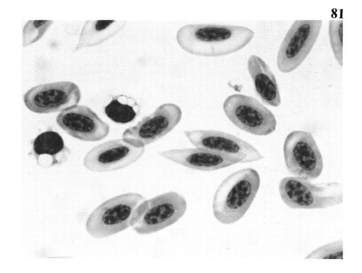

**81**

**82** A red cell showing basophilic stippling from a moose calf with slight hypochromic anaemia (Hb 10.0 g/dl). This is not an unusual finding in immature Artiodactyla and appears to be of no pathological significance.

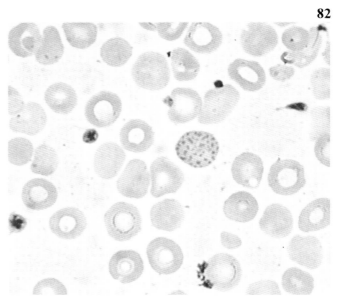

**82**

**83** Echinocytes and a polychromatic erythroblast from a giant anteater suffering from severe, regenerative haemorrhagic anaemia (Hb 2.1 g/dl).

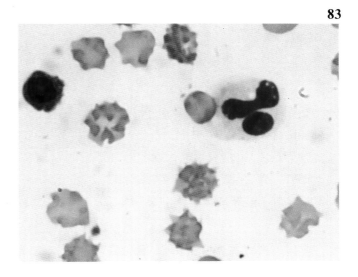

**83**

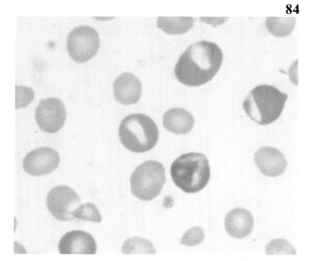

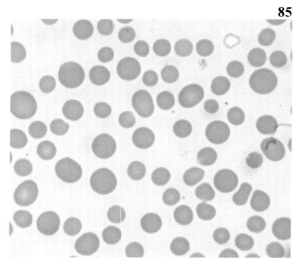

**84** Red cells showing polychromasia anisocytosis, poikilocytosis and stomatocytosis from a European hamster with moderately severe regenerative anaemia (Hb 6.7 g/dl).

**85** Marked anisocytosis in a domestic goat during recovery from severe haemorrhagic anaemia. The macrocytes are the newly formed cells. Polychromasia is not evident and the reticulocyte count was only slightly increased. Like many other ungulates, reticulocytes of goats do not enter the bloodstream in significant numbers, even after massive blood loss. In these animals, the presence of macrocytes is a more reliable indicator than the reticulocyte count of active erythropoiesis.

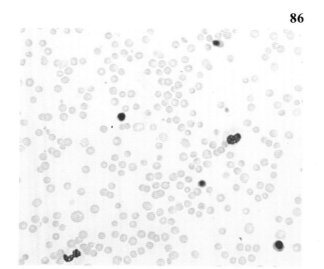

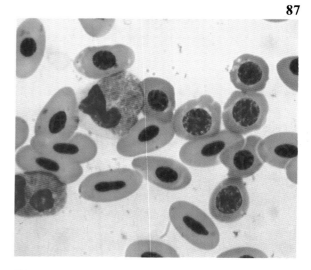

**86** Anisocytosis and erythroblasts in a cow with pyelonephritis and pyuria/haematuria (×40). This animal had neutrophilia with a left shift.

**87** Regenerative anaemia in a sarus crane. Four polychromatic erythroblasts and two normal heterophils are present.

**88** Four basophilic erythroblasts from a sacred ibis with moderately severe, regenerative anaemia associated with chronic infection (Hb 7.7 g/dl). The red cells show anisocytosis and some poikilocytosis.

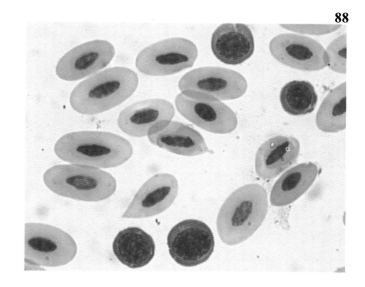

**89** Abnormal erythropoiesis in a golden eagle with severe regenerative anaemia, cause unknown (×40, Hb 5.1 g/dl).

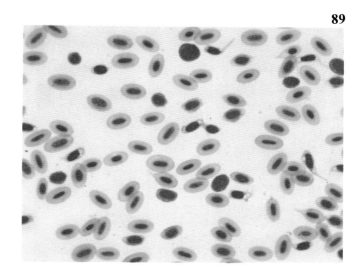

**90** Microcytic erythroblasts and an erythroblast in mitosis from the eagle in **89**. Two thrombocytes are present.

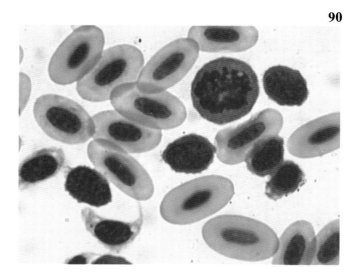

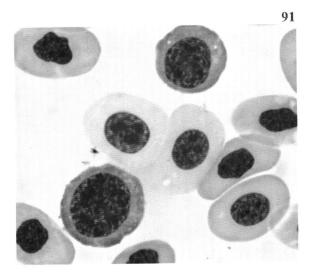

**91** Two basophilic erythroblasts from a gila monster (Hb 8.1 g/dl). One of these cells appears to be megaloblastic.

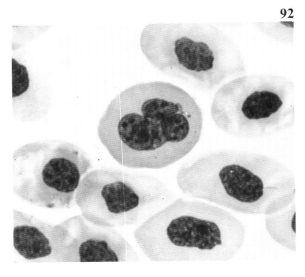

**92** A polychromatic megaloblast with abnormal nuclear division from the gila monster in **91**.

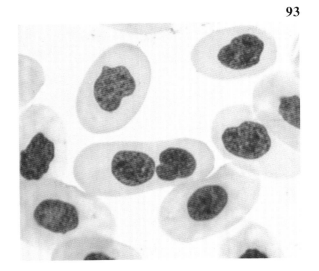

**93** A binucleated macrocyte and mature red cells with abnormal nuclei from the gila monster in **91**.

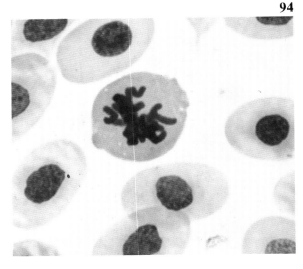

**94** A cell in mitosis, probably a polychromatic erythroblast, from the gila monster in **91**.

**95-98** *Erythropoiesis in a Mediterranean spur-thighed tortoise which had recently wakened from hibernation. This animal was slightly anaemic (Hb 6.2 g/l).*

**95**

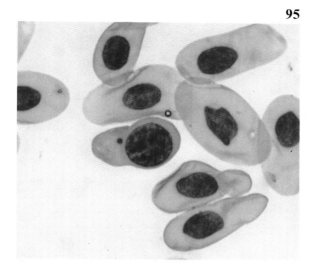

**95** A polychromatic erythroblast showing evidence of abnormal nuclear division. Several of the mature cells have folded cytoplasm.

**96**

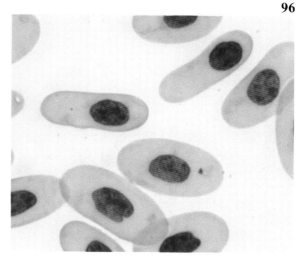

**96** Two red cells with asymmetrically placed nuclei and a cell with a small nuclear (?) fragment in the cytoplasm.

**97**

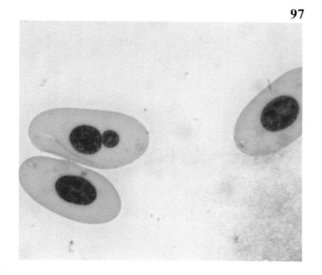

**97** A cell containing a large nuclear remnant (Howell Jolly body?).

**98**

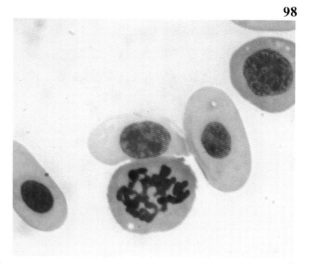

**98** A normal erythroblast and an erythroblast in mitosis.

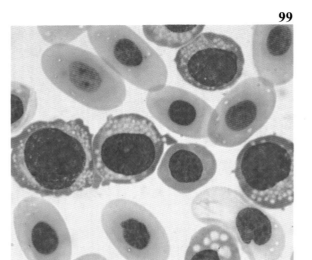

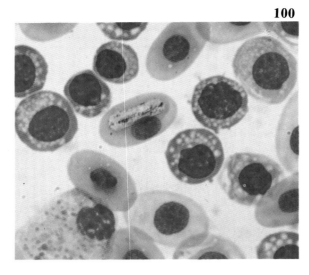

**99** Abnormal ( megaloblastic?) erythropoiesis in a Mediterranean spur-thighed tortoise suffering from anaemia and post-hibernation anorexia (Hb 3.2 g/dl).

**100** Basophilic and polychromatic erythroblasts with vacuolated cytoplasm from the tortoise in **99**. The red cell in the centre of the field contains a haemogregarine parasite which is thought to be non-pathogenic. There is a toxic heterophil at the bottom of the field.

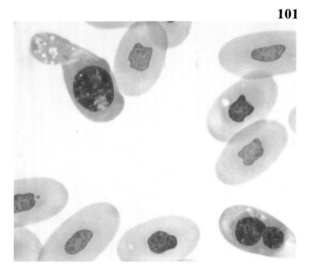

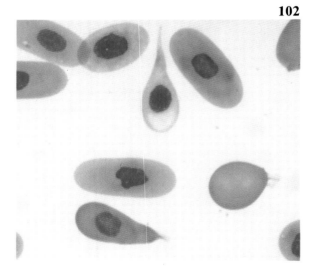

**101** Abnormal polychromatic erythroblasts from a boa constrictor suffering from chronic weight loss (Hb 6.7 g/dl).

**102** Two poikilocytes and an erythroplastid from the snake in **101**.

**103-106** *Autoimmune haemolytic anaemia in dogs.*

**103**

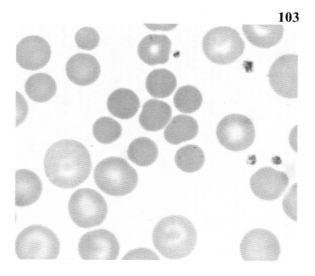

**103** Microspherocytes, target cells, anisocytosis and polychromasia. In this case, the presence of polychromatic red cells indicates active red cell replacement.

**104**

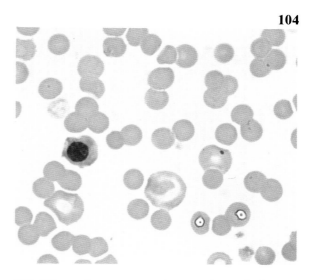

**104** Microspherocytes, anisocytosis, polychromasia, Howell Jolly bodies, agglutination and an orthochromic erythroblast. This case also shows active red cell replacement.

**105**

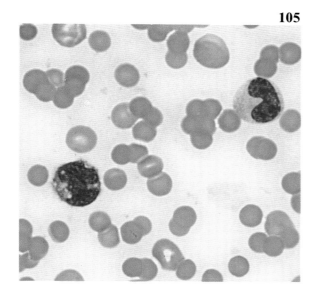

**105** Microspherocytes, anisocytosis, agglutination, a monocyte with vacuolated cytoplasm and a band neutrophil.

**106**

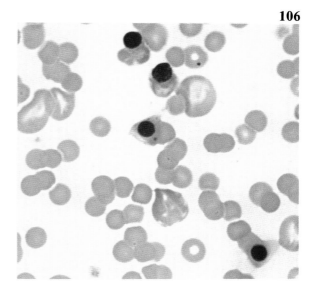

**106** Microspherocytes, anisocytosis, agglutination, polychromasia and two polychromatic and two orthochromic erythroblasts. The erythroblasts appear abnormal.

**107** Autoimmune haemolytic anaemia in a two-month-old wolf cub (Hb 9.8 g/dl). Microspherocytes, anisocytosis and an orthochromic erythroblast can be seen.

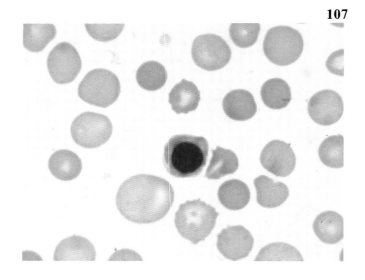

**108** Autoagglutination and marked polychromasia in a cat with warm agglutinin disease (×40).

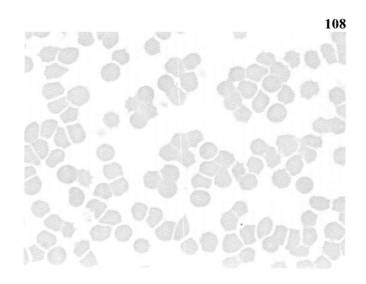

**109** Profound reticulocytosis in a cat with Coombs' positive regenerative anaemia (×40, new methylene blue stain). The cat was also Feline leukaemia virus (FeLV)-positive.

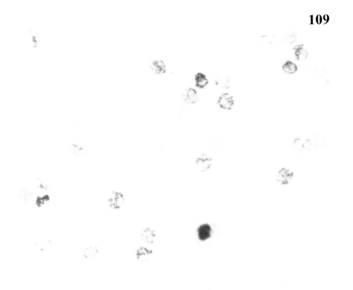

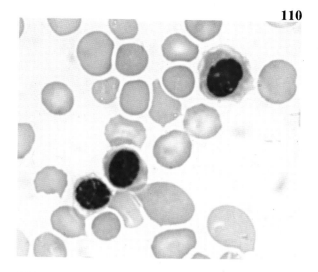

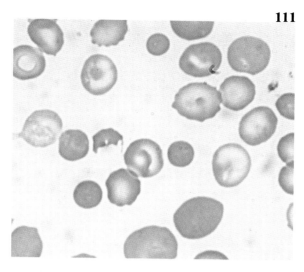

**110** Severe, regenerative haemolytic anaemia in a female ring-tailed coati (Hb 4.5 g/dl). The red cells show spherocytosis and anisocytosis. Three erythroblasts and several target cells are present.

**111** Marked anisocytosis, hypochromia, polychromasia, microspherocytes, schistocytes and target cells in the coati in **110**.

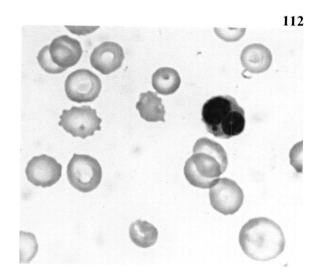

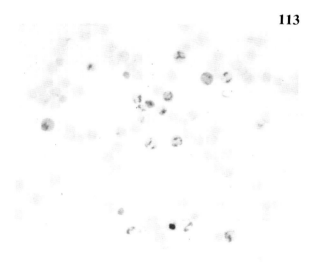

**112** A binucleated erythroblast from the coati in **110**.

**113** Marked reticulocytosis in the coati in **110** (×40, new methylene blue stain).

**114**

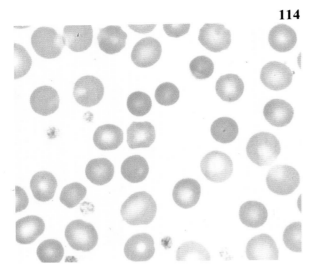

**114** Microspherocytes from a black spider monkey with peritonitis associated with chronic amoebiasis (Hb 9.8 g/dl).

**115**

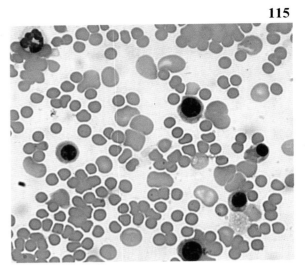

**115** Severe, regenerative haemolytic anaemia associated with necrobacillosis in a red-necked wallaby (×40, Hb 6.4 g/dl). The red cells show anisocytosis and autoagglutination and a large number of erythroblasts are present.

**116**

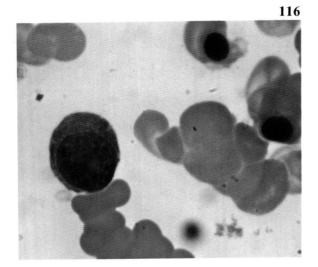

**116** A basophilic erythroblast and marked agglutination in the wallaby in **115**.

**117**

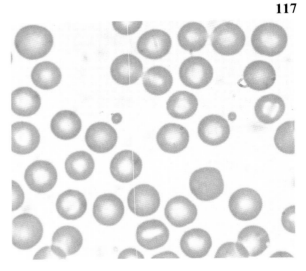

**117** Two extremely small microspherocytes from a tree shrew suffering from hypervitaminosis A.

**118** Red cell agglutination in an anaemic African grey parrot (Hb 8.4 g/dl). In this case the agglutination was caused by an antibody active at low temperatures and the bird was thought to have autoimmune haemolytic anaemia.

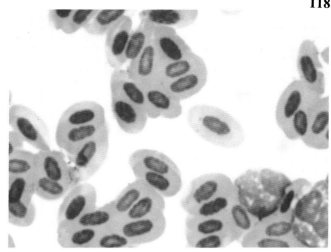

**119** Agglutinated red cells from the parrot in **118**, visible in a haemocytometer (×40, phase contrast microscopy).

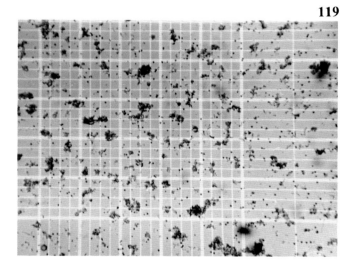

**120** Autoagglutination, similar to **119**, in an anaemic lesser sulphur-crested cockatoo (×40, Hb 9.0 g/dl).

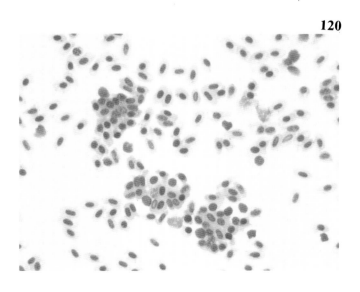

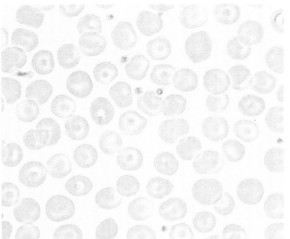

**121** Target cells from a dog.

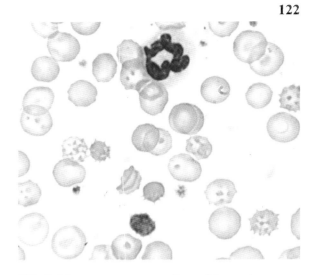

**122** Echinocytes, target cells and hypochromia in a hog badger with anaemia (Hb 6.9 g/dl). The animal was suffering from liver failure and toxaemia secondary to infected burns.

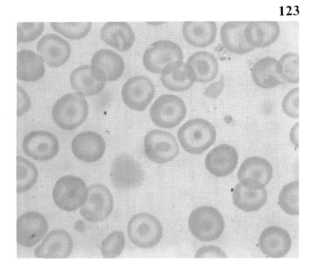

**123** Target cells and hypochromia in a prairie marmot with hypochromic anaemia (Hb 10.0 g/dl). The presence of target cells suggested that liver failure was present.

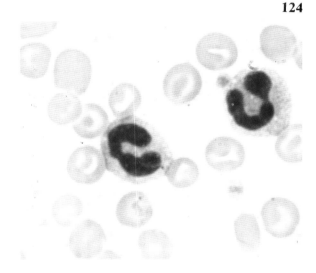

**124** Target cells and stomatocytes in a cotton-top tamarin with peritonitis (Hb 7.3 g/dl). Two neutrophils with reduced nuclear lobulation are present.

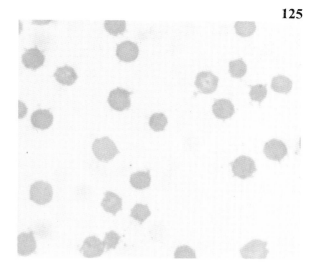

**125** Echinocytes from an Indian brown mongoose with slight non-regenerative normochromic anaemia secondary to kidney failure. The cause of the anaemia was probably depressed erythropoietin production.

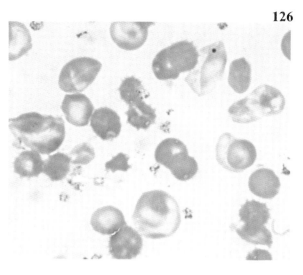

**126** Anisocytosis, poikilocytosis, hypochromasia and stomatocytosis in a ring-tailed coati with moderate non-regenerative anaemia associated with chronic infection (Hb 7.6 g/dl).

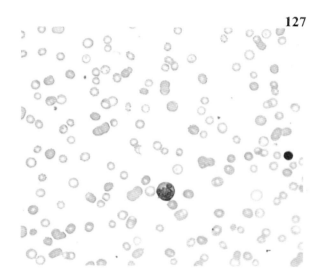

**127** Poikilocytes and schistocytes from a dog with endocarditis (×25).

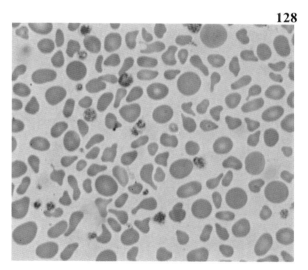

**128** Misshapen red cells from a newborn goat. The larger, discoid cells are presumed to contain adult haemoglobin. The relative number of these increased progressively with time.

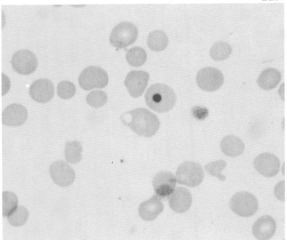

**129** Severe regenerative anaemia in a 5-day-old roan antelope calf (Hb 6.2 g/dl). The red cells show anisocytosis. One large Howell Jolly body is present and one cell appears to have a hole at the periphery.

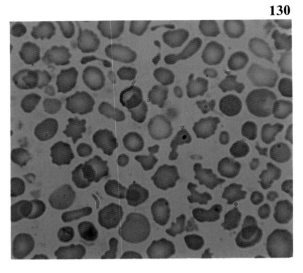

**130** Extreme red cell deformation in a 1-day-old roan antelope calf (Hb 10.1 g/dl). Cells of this type frequently occur in the blood of immature ungulates and appear to be associated with a high neonatal mortality rate. In animals which survive, the abnormal cells are progressively replaced by normal biconcave discocytes containing adult haemoglobin. Unlike sickled red cells, this type of red cell shape abnormality cannot be reversed by altering the conditions in the blood sample.

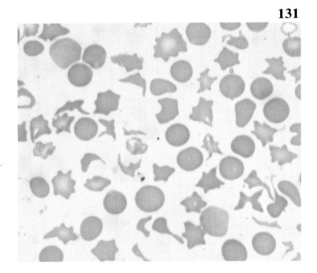

**131** Extreme red cell deformation and some normal red cells in a severely ill, 1-day-old Arabian oryx calf.

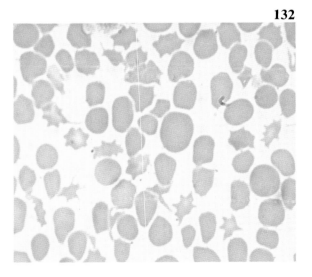

**132** Two morphologically distinct populations of red cells in a 10-week-old gaur calf. More than 50 per cent of the cells appear normal and are presumed to be those produced in the post-natal period. The presence of macrocytes indicates active erythropoiesis. This animal was not anaemic (Hb 18.0 g/dl).

**133** Blood film from a 25-day-old scimitar-horned oryx calf showing similar red cell deformation (Hb 7.1 g/dl). Some apparently normal cells are present.

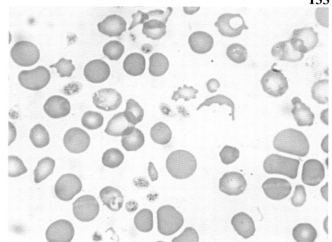

**134** SEM of the sample in **133** showing evidence that an early stage in the development of the misshapen red cells is the appearance of holes in some of the cells. Progressive increase in the size of the holes and eventual rupture of the cells containing them could result in the bizarre cell shapes observed.

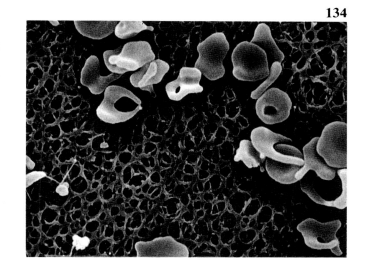

**135** Blood film from the scimitar-horned oryx in **133** at the age of 7 weeks (Hb 10.1 g/dl). A larger proportion of normal red cells is present.

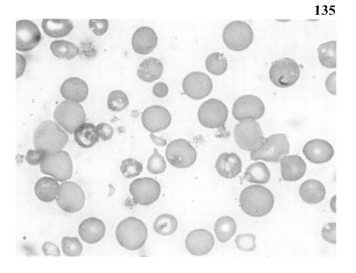

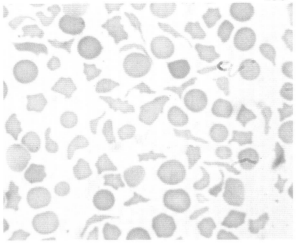

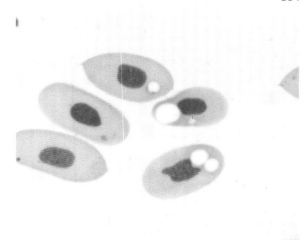

**136** Misshapen red cells in an 8-week-old fallow deer fawn (Hb 13.1 g/dl). A few sickle cells are also present; these revert to normal biconcave discs when deoxygenated.

**137** Vacuolated red cells from a royal python with chronic weight loss (Hb 6.0 g/dl). Red cell vacuolation is not unusual in normal snakes of this group. One of the red cells has a misshapen nucleus. This finding appears to be associated with malnutrition in reptiles.

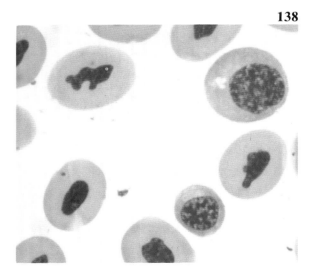

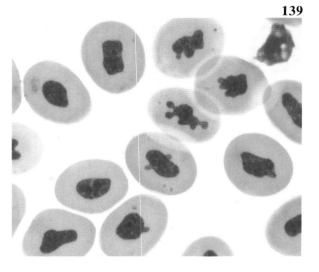

**138** A macrocytic and a microcytic polychromatic erythroblast from a boomslang with anorexia and necrotic stomatitis. The animal was not anaemic (Hb 13.3 g/dl) but the red cell nuclei were deformed.

**139** Red cells from the boomslang in **138** with marked nuclear deformation and the budding off of small Howell Jolly body-like fragments.

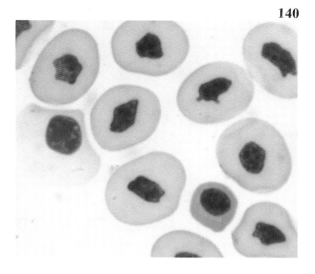

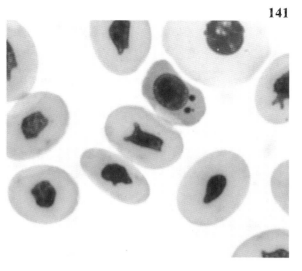

**140** Red cells with misshapen nuclei from a hawksbill turtle suffering from malnutrition (Hb 10.6 g/dl).

**141** A polychromatic erythroblast showing evidence of abnormal nuclear division from the turtle in **140**.

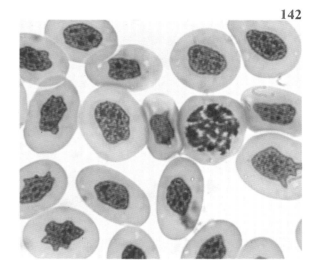

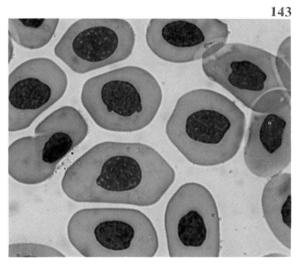

**142** Red cells with misshapen nuclei from a blue-tongued skink with chronic infection and anorexia (Hb 6.7 g/dl). The red cell nuclei appear megaloblastic. A polychromatic erythroblast in mitosis is present.

**143** Anisocytosis in an Aldabra giant tortoise suffering from malnutrition and anaemia (Hb 5.2 g/dl). Some of the cells are less elliptical than normal and the nuclei show signs of immaturity.

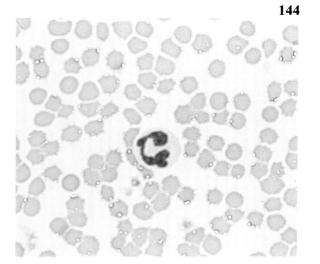

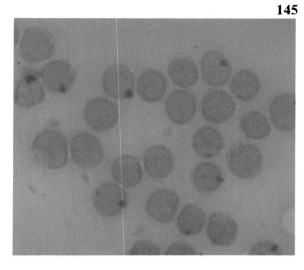

**144** Erythrocyte refractile (ER) bodies in an unstained blood film from a cat suffering from paracetamol intoxication. ER bodies are analagous with Heinz bodies.

**145** Red cells from the cat in **144** with paracetamol intoxication, stained supravitally with new methylene blue to show the Heinz bodies.

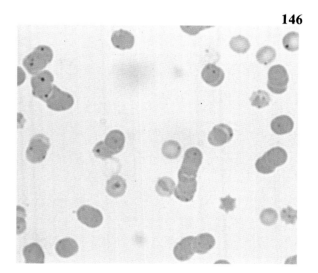

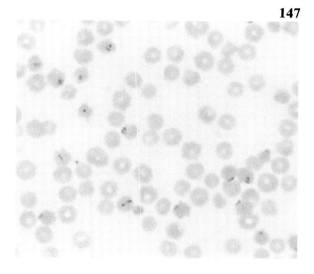

**146** *Haemobartonella felis* and Howell Jolly bodies in red cells from a cat (×40).

**147** Multiple *Babesia divergens* in red cells from a Fresian cow.

**148** Increased rouleaux formation in a dog with myeloma.

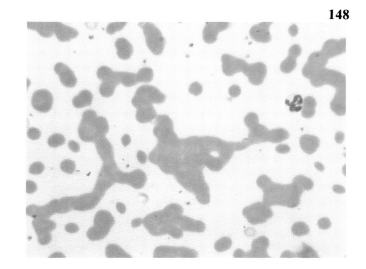

**149** Increased rouleaux formation in a dog with neoplasia. A normal neutrophil and two neutrophils with decreased nuclear lobulation (left shift) and abnormal cytoplasmic granules are present.

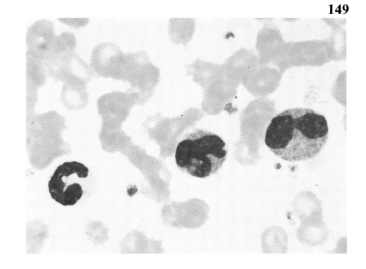

**150** Bone marrow preparation from a dog with polycythaemia vera rubra.

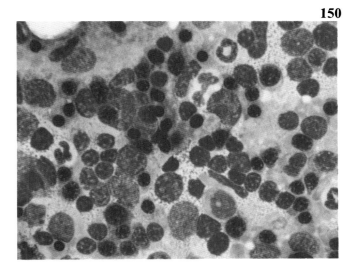

# Part 2
# Normal and Abnormal Granulocytes

The classification of white blood cells and the identification of morphological abnormalities on stained blood films depends not only upon observation of differences in the form and size of the nucleus and cytoplasm but also upon the staining characteristics of the cell constituents. The stains most widely used for this purpose are Romanowsky stains. These contain azure complexes which react with acidic groupings, including those of nucleic acids and proteins of the cell nuclei and primitive cytoplasm, and eosin Y which has an affinity for the basic groupings on haemoglobin and other molecules. Several different varieties of Romanowsky stain are available, each of which produces slightly different results. All are suitable for comparative work; the choice is a matter of personal preference. It should be recognised, however, that these stains are difficult to standardise, even when used on a single species. When applied to a range of species, the variations seen may result from uncontrolled staining differences as well as from true species diversity. In addition, the morphology of the cells and the way in which they take up the stains can be modified by technical factors such as the anticoagulant used, improper drying of the cells on the slide, prolonged storage or inadequate fixation.

White cells with granular cytoplasm occur in the blood of all mammals, birds and reptiles. Mammalian granulocytes are classified as neutrophils, eosinophils and basophils on the strength of the reaction of their cytoplasmic granules with Romanowsky stains. This classification is largely descriptive and originates from observations on the reactions of human white cells with Romanowsky stains. In normal human blood, the neutrophil granules are relatively small and stain weakly with the azure complexes; the basophil granules are larger, spherical, completely fill the cytoplasm and react strongly with the azure complexes; the eosinophil granules are round, numerous and have an affinity for eosin. Changes in the staining characteristics and distribution of the granules can be of diagnostic significance.

Among other mammals, the granulocyte nuclei are polymorphic in all species although there is much species variation in the degree of lobulation and in the number of lobes normally present. There is also species variation in the size, shape, distribution and staining characteristics of the cytoplasmic granules, particularly those of the neutrophils. Neutrophil granules can be basophilic as, for example, in chimpanzees and some artiodactyls, or strongly eosinophilic as in rabbits and some rodents. In some species, the cytoplasm of these cells appears agranular or contains only faint pink particles. In these animals, the cells are classified as neutrophil granulocytes on the strength of their polymorphic (lobed) nuclei and on the absence of specific eosinophilic or basophilic granules. The granules of the eosinophils and basophils can also show species variation in size, number, shape and staining intensity. The cytoplasm of eosinophils, if visible, usually appears pale blue.

The same three types of granulocyte can be distinguished in the blood of birds and reptiles and, although there are differences in morphology and terminology, it is probable that the cells are functionally similar to those of mammals. The terminological difference stems from the fact that the cells of birds and reptiles which are generally assumed to be homologous with mammalian neutrophils have cytoplasm containing a large number of strongly eosinophilic, usually spiculate or oval granules. The term 'neutrophil,' therefore, is not appropriate and these cells are generally known as heterophils. In reptiles, a further cell type, the azurophil, is found. Although azurophils are considered by some haematologists to represent neutrophil granulocytes, they have been included with other mononuclear cells in Part 3 (page 107).

The heterophils of birds show little interspecies variation and characteristically have a lobed, usually bilobed, nucleus and spiculate or oval granules which stain brick red with Romanowsky stains and usually fill the cytoplasm. If visible, the cytoplasm appears colourless or faintly pink. In contrast to those of birds, reptilian heterophils show considerable morphological diversity. In the Serpentes (snakes), Crocodylia (crocodiles and alligators) and Testudines (tortoises, turtles and terrapins), they are large cells with an unlobed, round or oval, often excentric nucleus and spiculate granules which fill the cytoplasm. The granules stain bright orange/red in lizards, snakes and chelonians and brick red in crocodilians. In some species of Sauria (lizards), the heterophil nucleus is round and in others it is lobed and resembles that of birds.

Neutrophil/heterophil granulocytes are the most numerous of the granulocytes found in normal mammals, birds and reptiles. Their primary function is bacterial killing, involving chemotaxis, opsonisation, ingestion and lysis. An increase in the number of these cells in the circulating blood occurs in response to bacterial and fungal infections, tissue damage, some metabolic diseases, myeloid leukaemias and stress. There are marked species differences in the quantitative response detectable in the peripheral blood and morphological variation can often be more informative than absolute cell counts.

In birds and reptiles, the presence of eosinophilic granules in the heterophils gives rise to problems in distinguishing between these cells and the true eosinophils. Further problems can result from inadequate fixation which results in degranulation of the heterophils and basophils. In practice, avian and reptilian heterophils and eosinophils can usually be differentiated by the appearance of their granules. Heterophil granules are usually spiculate or oval and, in birds, stain with a brick-red colour, whereas the granules of true eosinophils are usually round and stain a clear bright red. If visible, the cytoplasm of the heterophils is colourless or pale pink and that of the eosinophils is blue.

Marrow biopsy for diagnostic purposes is not often feasible in sick animals but, since immature granulocytes are rarely found in the bloodstream of healthy individuals, their presence on a peripheral blood film is a valuable indication of increased demand or marrow dysfunction and it is important to recognise these cells when they occur. Granulopoiesis has been studied extensively in man and in some other mammals and, although less is known about the subject in birds and reptiles, it appears that the process is essentially similar in all three groups. The earliest recognisable cell of the granulocyte series is the myeloblast (granuloblast) which gives rise to promyelocytes (progranulocytes), myelocytes, metamyelocytes and mature granulocytes in sequence. Succeeding maturation stages are differentiated on the basis of progressive decrease in cell size and cytoplasmic basophilia, condensation and, in mammals and birds, segmentation of the nucleus and the appearance of an increasing complement of specific cytoplasmic granules. Difficulties can arise from the fact that there is a transient appearance of basophilic granules in avian and reptilian heterophil myelocytes and metamyelocytes which may lead to confusion between these cells and mature basophils. Additional problems in distinguishing between heterophils and eosinophils can arise from the fact that the eosinophilic granules in immature avian heterophils are spherical as opposed to rod-shaped. Thus, there is a possibility for confusion of immature cells of the heterophil series with both basophils and eosinophils.

## THE BLOOD FILM

The most usefully observed morphological changes affecting neutrophils and heterophils are those which reflect immaturity or toxicity. The presence in the circulating blood of immature granulocytes is a valuable indicator of myeloid hyperplasia associated with either malignancy or infectious and other inflammatory conditions. In some species, the neutrophil/heterophil response to inflammation is qualitative rather than quantitative and, in these animals, the finding of cells showing signs of immaturity is a more reliable index of increased demand as, for example, in bacterial infection, than is the total white cell count. Information about the stage of maturity of the neutrophils is also important for distinguishing between disease and stress-induced neutrophilia. Immature granulocytes can be identified from their larger size, cytoplasmic basophilia and lack of specific granules. In animals in which the neutrophil/heterophil nuclei are normally lobed, immaturity is further characterised by a decrease in number or absence of nuclear lobes (left shift). In reptiles in which the heterophil nucleus is normally round, lobulation can be an indication of infection. The presence of increased basophilia, toxic granules, Döhle bodies and/or vacuoles in the cytoplasm can also be of diagnostic significance. Some of these criteria, for example, the finding of metamyelocytes and their precursors or cells containing Döhle bodies or cytoplasmic vacuoles, should be applicable to all species; pathological variations in nuclear lobulation and cytoplasmic granulation, however, may not be recognised without reference to normal cells of the species concerned.

**151-222** *Species variation in normal granulocytes.*

**151**

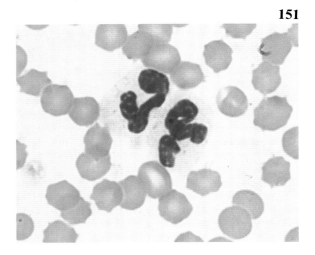

**151** Two neutrophils with agranular cytoplasm and indistinct nuclear lobulation from a jaguar. These cells are typical of the neutrophils found in feline animals.

**152**

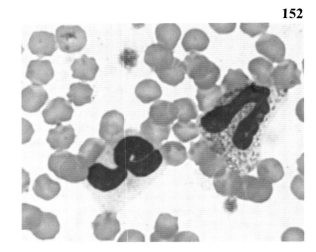

**152** An agranular neutrophil and an eosinophil with small red cytoplasmic granules from a domestic cat. The nuclear lobes are poorly defined in both cells.

**153**

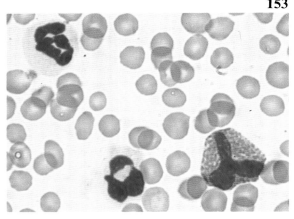

**153** Two agranular neutrophils and an eosinophil from a cheetah (×40).

**154**

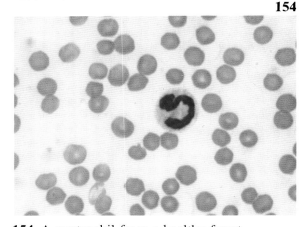

**154** A neutrophil from a healthy ferret.

**155**

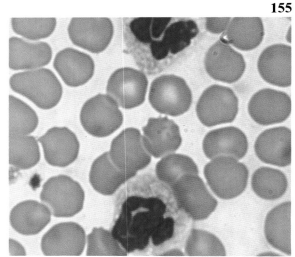

**155** Two neutrophils from a polar bear. The cytoplasm contains aggregates of pink-staining material and the nuclear lobes are well defined.

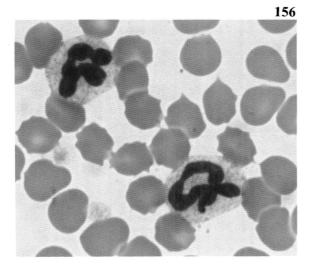

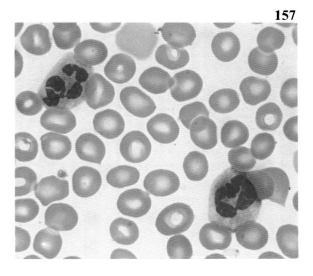

**156** Two neutrophils from a healthy dog. The cells have faint, pink, cytoplasmic granules.

**157** Two neutrophils from a healthy human individual.

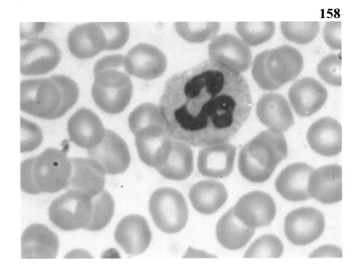

**158** A neutrophil with pink granules and well-defined nuclear lobes from an orang utan.

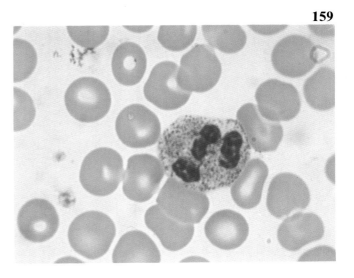

**159** A chimpanzee neutrophil with some basophilic granules.

**160** A neutrophil with orange-staining granules and a relatively large number of well-defined nuclear lobes from a white-headed saki monkey. The neutrophils of Old World monkeys tend to have a greater number of lobes than those of man.

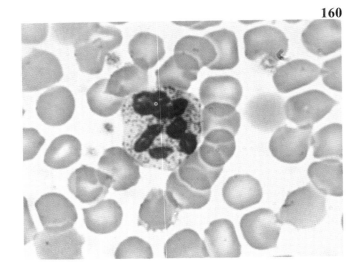

**161** Two neutrophils from a healthy rhesus macaque.

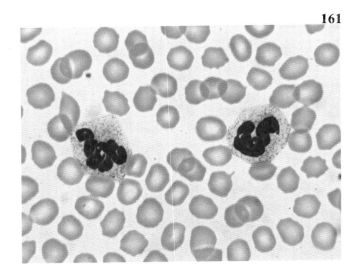

**162** A neutrophil and a lymphocyte from a healthy cynomolgus (crab-eating) macaque.

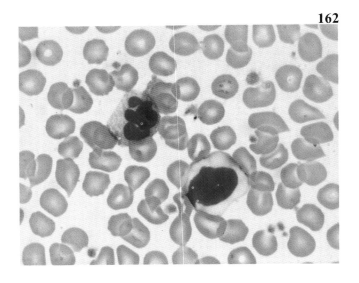

**163** Two neutrophils with many orange and a few purple granules and an eosinophil with indistinct red granules from a healthy owl monkey.

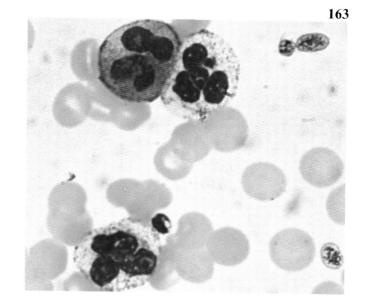

**163**

**164** Two neutrophils and a lymphocyte from a healthy common marmoset.

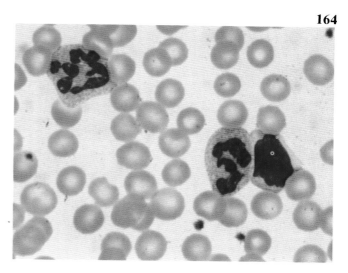

**164**

**165** A neutrophil and an eosinophil from a brown lemur. These cells have staining characteristics similar to those of the owl monkey.

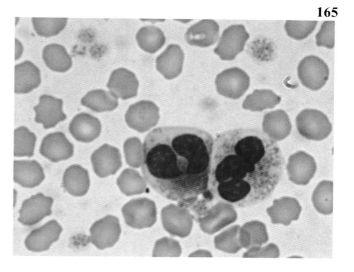

**165**

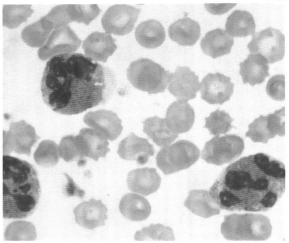

**166** Three neutrophils with strongly eosinophilic cytoplasmic granules from a rabbit. These cells are sometimes known as 'pseudoeosinophils' and can be confused with true eosinophils.

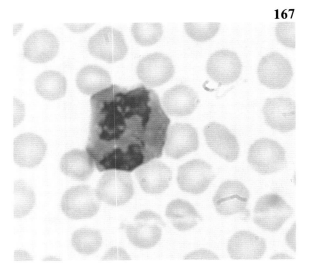

**167** Comparison with a true eosinophil from the rabbit in **166**. The eosinophils have larger, more numerous and somewhat poorly defined, eosinophilic granules, some of which may overlie the nucleus. The nucleus usually has fewer lobes than that of the 'pseudoeosinophil'.

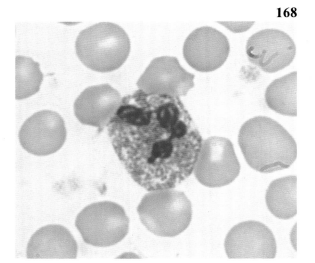

**168** A 'pseudoeosinophilic' neutrophil from a capybara. The neutrophil granules of many hystricomorph rodents show these staining characteristics.

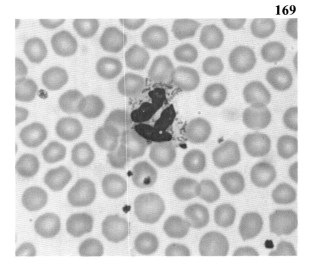

**169** A 'pseudoeosinophilic' neutrophil from a healthy guinea pig.

**170** A neutrophil with agranular cytoplasm and a ring-form nucleus from a mouse. Compared with hystriocomorph and sciuromorph rodents, the nuclei of myomorph rodent neutrophils have poorly defined lobes.

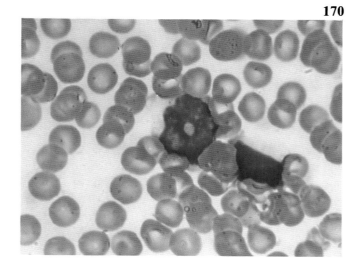

**170**

**171** A neutrophil from a healthy rat. The nuclear lobes are poorly defined and there are small, pale pink cytoplasmic granules. The red cells are crenated.

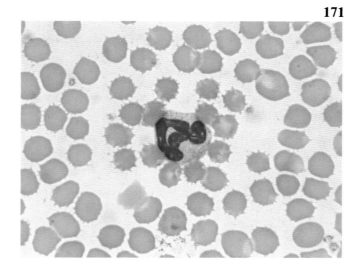

**171**

**172** A neutrophil with a multilobed nucleus (right shift) and a normal lymphocyte from a healthy grey squirrel.

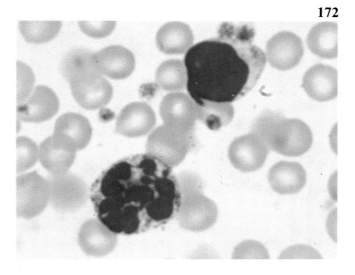

**172**

**173** A neutrophil with small basophilic granules and distinct nuclear lobes from a roan antelope. The red cells are crenated.

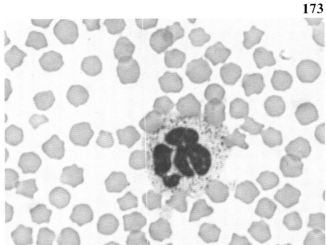

**174** A neutrophil from a moose with similar characteristics to the antelope in **173**.

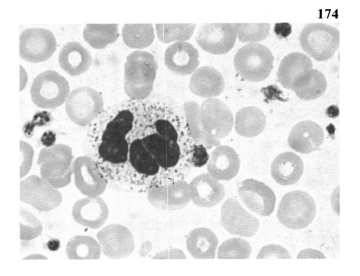

**175** An agranular neutrophil from a domestic cow.

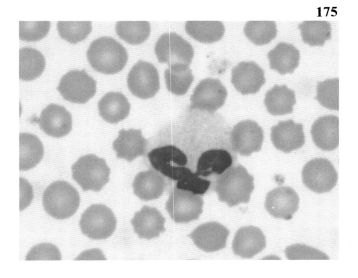

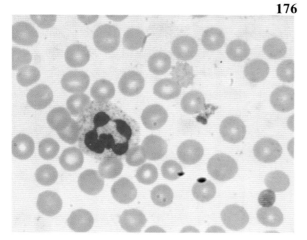

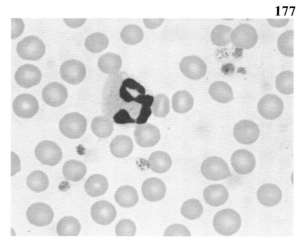

**176** A neutrophil from a healthy eland. The cell is indistinguishable from those of domestic cattle.

**177** A neutrophil from a yak.

**178** A neutrophil with a condensed nucleus with a drumstick appendage from a female common hippopotamus. The red cells show marked crenation.

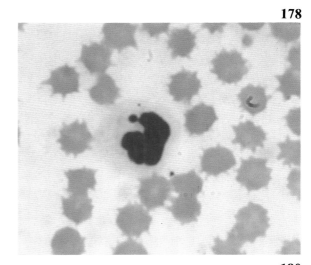

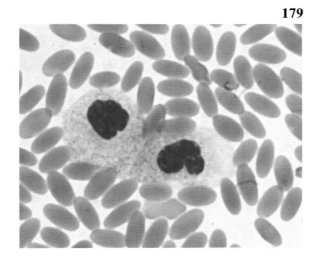

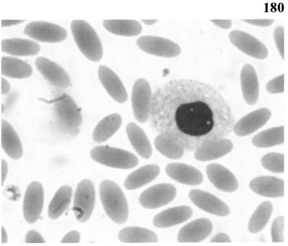

**179, 180** Neutrophils with condensed, bilobed or unlobed nuclei from bactrian camels. The appearance of the nuclei is similar to that seen in humans, dogs, cats and rabbits showing the Pelger-Huët phenomenon. Neutrophils of this type occur in some but not all bactrian camels. Possible patterns of inheritance have not yet been studied. There is no evidence of associated impairment of cell function.

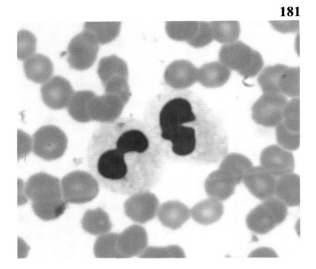

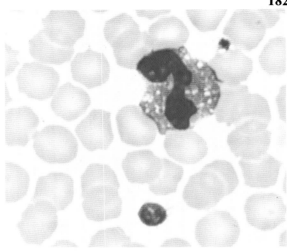

**181** Two neutrophils showing a Pelger-Huët-like phenomenon from a white rhinoceros. As in bactrian camels, these cells are found in some but not all individuals of the species and appear to function normally.

**182** An eosinophil with cytoplasmic vacuoles from a dog (terrier). Cells of this type are normal in some canine breeds.

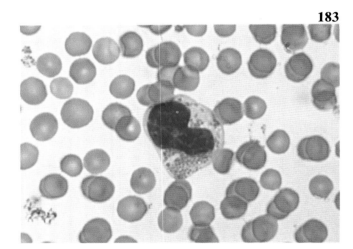

**183** An eosinophil with distinct, small eosinophilic granules which do not completely fill the blue/grey cytoplasm from a blesbok.

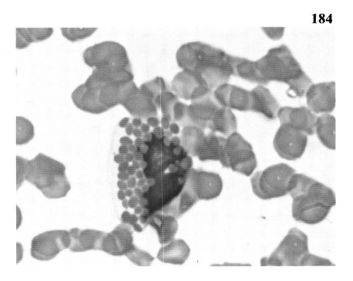

**184** An eosinophil from a horse. The cytoplasm is completely filled with large, spherical, strongly eosinophilic granules. A high degree of red cell rouleaux formation, as shown, is normal in horses.

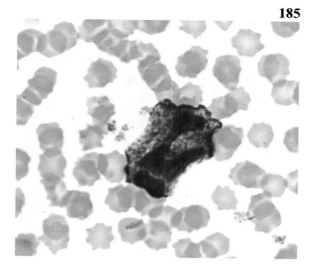

**185** A basophil from a gaur. The granules do not completely mask the lobed nucleus.

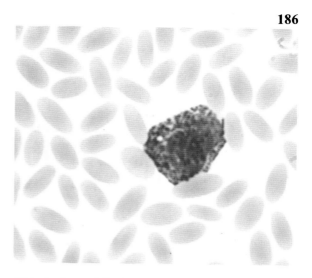

**186** A basophil from a bactrian camel. The granules show variation in staining intensity and do not mask the nucleus.

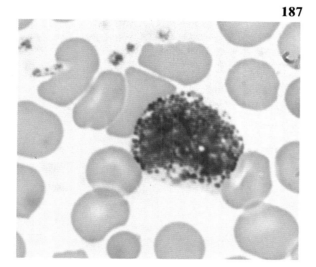

**187** A basophil with distinct spherical granules showing differences in staining density from a two-toed sloth. This species has comparatively large red cells.

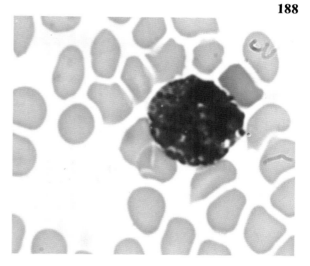

**188** A typical basophil from a guinea pig.

**189** In birds and reptiles, the cells analagous with mammalian neutrophils have strongly eosinophilic cytoplasmic granules and are known as heterophils. In some species, it can be difficult to distinguish between heterophils and eosinophils. In most birds, heterophils have brick red, oval or spiculate granules whereas the eosinophil granules are usually round and more brightly eosinophilic. A typical avian heterophil and eosinophil from a Javan fish owl are shown. The heterophil (top) has brick red, spiculate granules; the eosinophil has bright red, round granules. Both cells have bilobed nuclei.

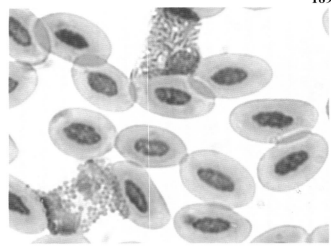

**190** A typical avian heterophil from a rosy flamingo.

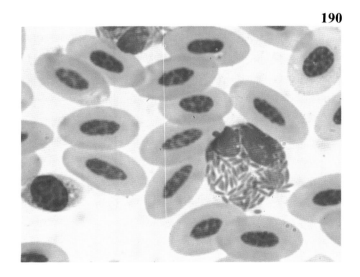

**191** Four heterophils from an apparently healthy domestic fowl. The nucleus of one of these cells shows decreased lobulation, suggesting sub-clinical inflammatory disease.

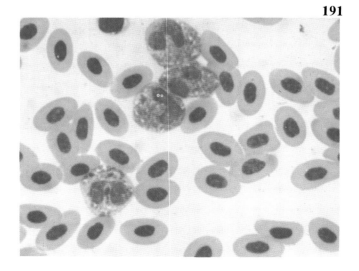

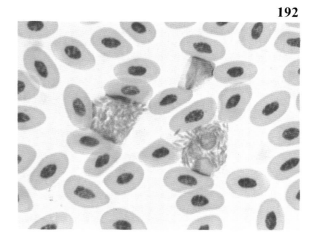

**192** Two heterophils and a lymphocyte from a domestic turkey.

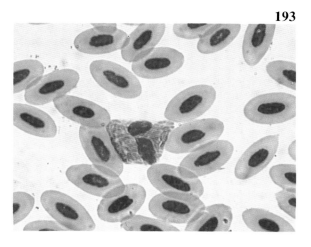

**193** A heterophil from a domestic goose.

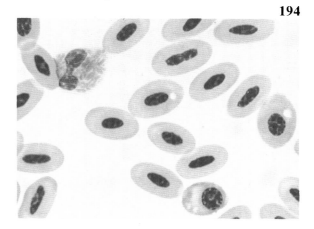

**194** A heterophil from a domestic duck. A polychromatic erythroblast is also present.

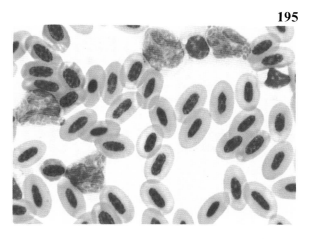

**195** Heterophils and two thrombocytes from a normal pigeon. The red cells show polychromasia.

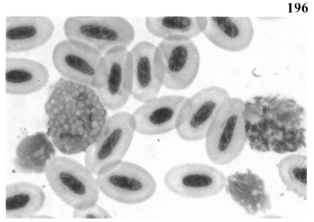

**196** A heterophil with indistinct brick red granules and an eosinophil with distinctive round, brighter red granules from a kori bustard. Both cells have bilobed nuclei. Two disrupted red cell nuclei are also present.

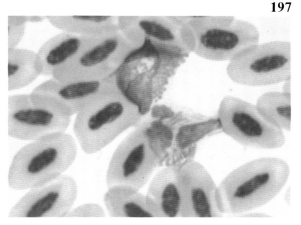

**197** A heterophil with indistinct, brick red, spiculate granules and an eosinophil with brighter red, spherical granules from a common buzzard. Both cells have bilobed nuclei.

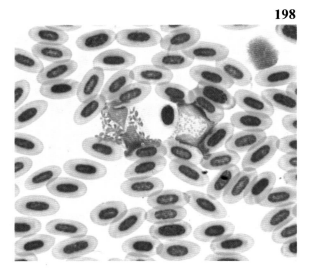 198

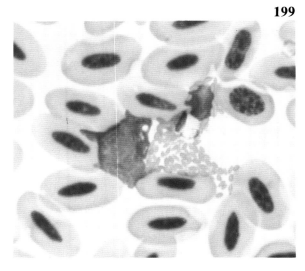 199

**198** A heterophil and an eosinophil from a healthy canary. The eosinophil has sparse, round, orange-staining cytoplasmic granules in contrast to those of the heterophil which are brick red and spiculate.

**199** An intact heterophil with brick red granules and a broken eosinophil with oval orange granules from a white stork.

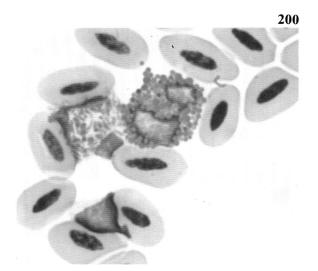 200

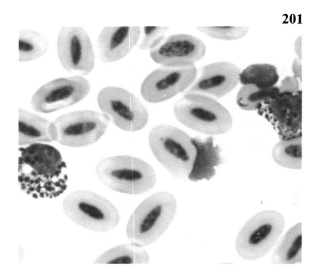 201

**200** A heterophil with typical brick red, spiculate granules and a trilobed nucleus, a slightly disrupted eosinophil with bluish, spherical granules and a bilobed nucleus from a lesser sulphurcrested cockatoo. The basophilic nature of the eosinophil granules is characteristic of most psittacine birds.

**201** Two normal basophils, for comparison, from the cockatoo in **200**.

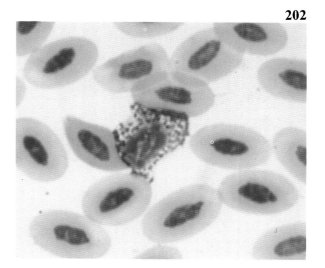

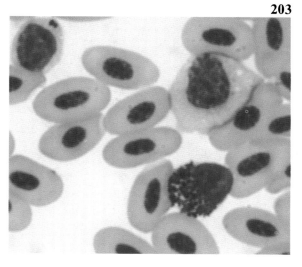

**202** A basophil with sparse purple granules from a Javan fish owl.

**203** A basophil with dark purple granules, a lymphocyte with a cytoplasmic granule (left) and a monocyte from a hooded crane.

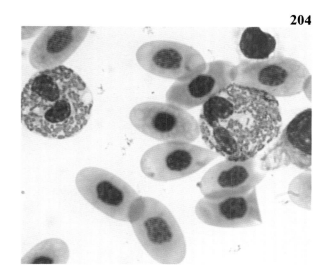

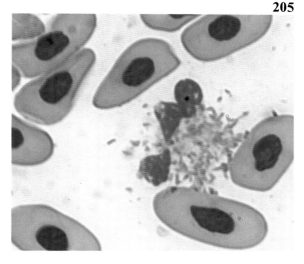

**204** Two heterophils from a healthy common iguana. The cells have bilobed nuclei and bacilliform, eosinophilic cytoplasmic granules and are somewhat similar to the heterophils found in birds. Heterophils with lobed nuclei occur in many but not all species of Sauria (lizards) whereas those of Testudines (tortoises, terrapins and turtles), Crocodylia (crocodiles and alligators) and Serpentes (snakes) have unlobed nuclei.

**205** A ruptured heterophil from the iguana in **204** showing the bacilliform eosinophilic granules and lobed nucleus.

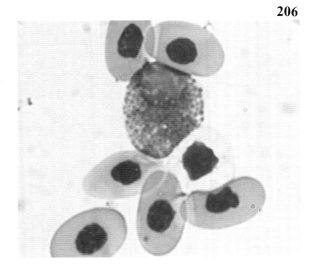

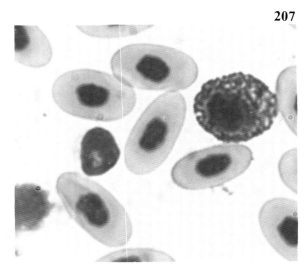

**206** An eosinophil from a healthy common iguana. Unlike the eosinophils of most other reptiles, these have round, bluish granules.

**207** A basophil, for comparison, from the iguana in **206**.

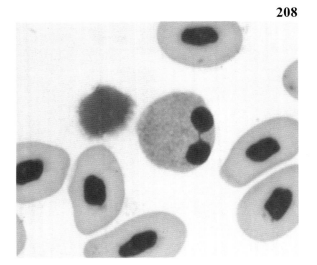

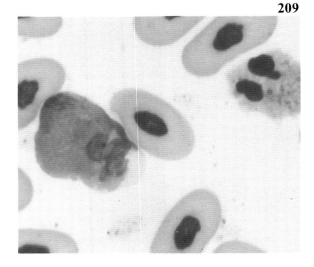

**208, 209** Cells with bilobed nuclei, resembling mammalian neutrophils, found occasionally in the blood of some species of Sauria, in this case a common iguana. The origin of these cells is not known; possibly they are necrotic granulocytes. A normal heterophil with coalescent granules is present in **209**.

**210** A heterophil from a plated lizard. The nucleus is bilobed.

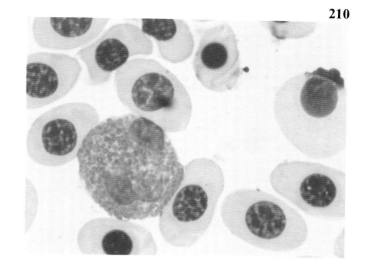

**211** A heterophil with a trilobed nucleus and a basophil completely filled with granules from a black-pointed tegu.

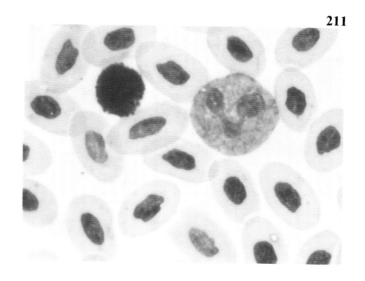

**212** Two heterophils with bilobed nuclei and sparse eosinophilic granules from a healthy shingleback skink. Cells of this type are typical of skinks.

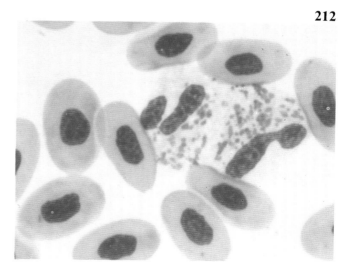

**213** A heterophil from a healthy Nile monitor lizard. Monitors and water dragons are examples of Sauria which have heterophils with unlobed nuclei, similar to those of Chelonia, Serpentes and Crocodylia.

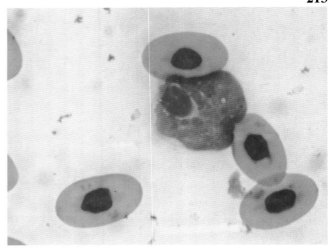

**214** A heterophil with an unlobed, excentric nucleus from a healthy Indian python. A polychromatic erythroblast with cytoplasmic vacuoles is also present.

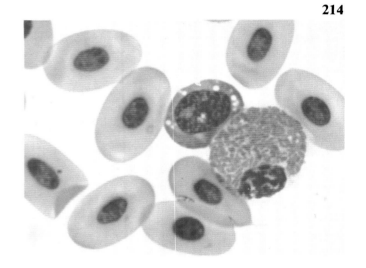

**215** A ruptured heterophil from a brown python showing the round nucleus and bacilliform eosinophilic granules. The cell on the left is an azurophil.

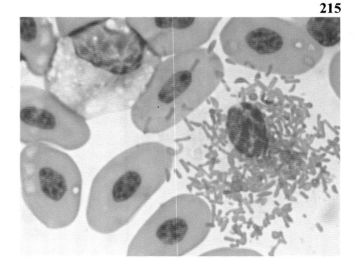

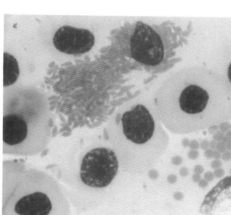

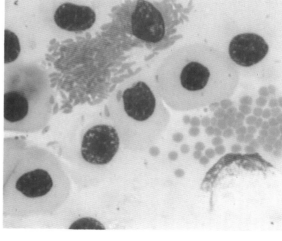

**216** A heterophil and an eosinophil from an Aldabra giant tortoise. The heterophil (left) has irregular, bacilliform, magenta-coloured granules, while those of the eosinophil are round and pale red. Both cells have unlobed nuclei.

**217** A ruptured heterophil and a ruptured eosinophil from a peacock soft-shelled turtle showing differences in granule shape and staining characteristics.

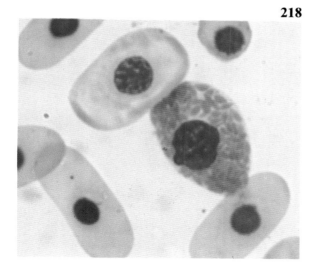

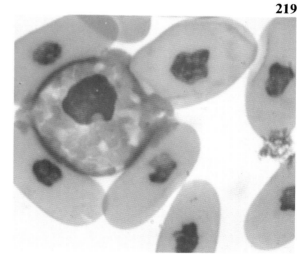

**218** A heterophil from a Mississippi alligator.

**219** An eosinophil from a Chinese alligator.

**220** An intact and a ruptured basophil from a boa constrictor. Both spiculate and round granules are present.

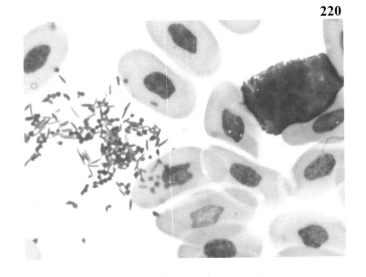

**221** The boa constrictor in **220**, showing granules from a ruptured basophil which, under some circumstances, might be mistaken for parasites, bacteria or red cell nuclear remnants.

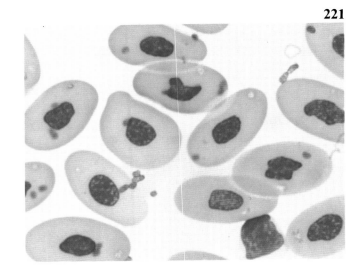

**222** Three basophils from a healthy red-eared terrapin. The morphological differences in the two intact cells may reflect different stages in maturation. Alternatively, it is possible that mast cells occur normally in the peripheral blood of some terrapins. The basophil is a relatively abundant cell in this species.

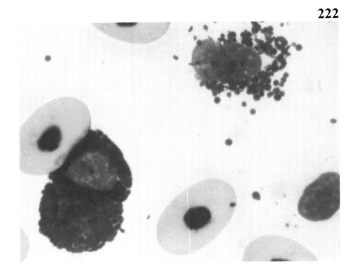

**223** Three degranulated heterophils in a blood film from a sarus crane. The cytoplasm contains irregular spaces surrounded by aggregations of eosinophilic material. This artefact is usually associated with inadequate fixation. The lobed nature of the heterophil nuclei is clearly evident. A disrupted red cell nucleus and a normal monocyte are also present.

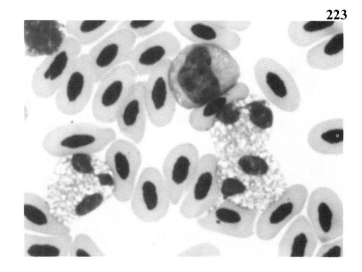

223

**224** Two degranulated heterophils in a poorly fixed blood film from an emu. The cytoplasm of one heterophil contains some bacilliform granules, a number of round vacuoles containing small round eosinophilic granules and areas of amorphous eosinophilic material. The second heterophil shows a more advanced degree of deterioration in that bacilliform granules are absent and the nucleus is degenerate.

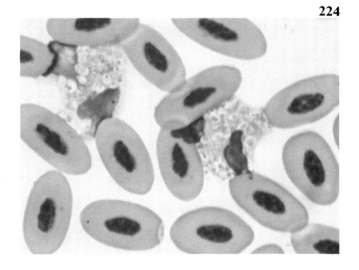

224

**225** A partially degranulated basophil from a sarus crane. Several disrupted red cell nuclei are present.

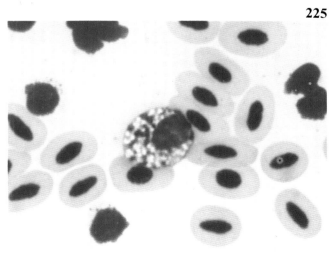

225

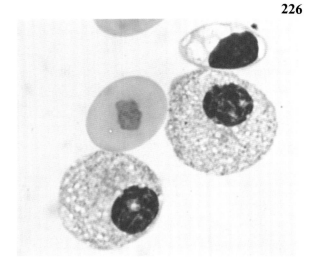

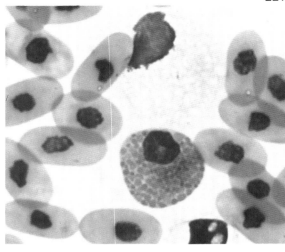

**226** Two degranulated heterophils and a normal thrombocyte from a Nile crocodile. The unlobed nature of the heterophil nuclei is clearly evident. The nuclei of the red cells are poorly stained.

**227** A disintegrating degranulated heterophil, a normal eosinophil and a normal thrombocyte from the crocodile in **226**.

**228** A degranulated heterophil from a gila monster. The adjacent small cell is a microcytic polychromatic normoblast.

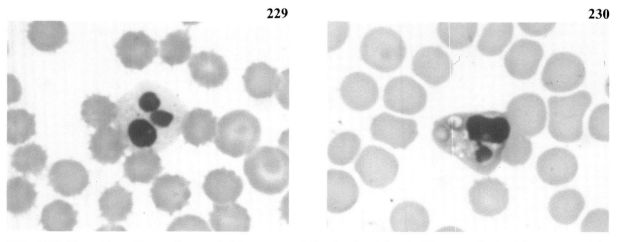

**229, 230** Necrotic white cells, probably neutrophils, in dog blood. The sample had been stored in EDTA for 24 hours.

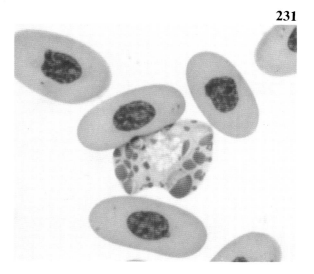

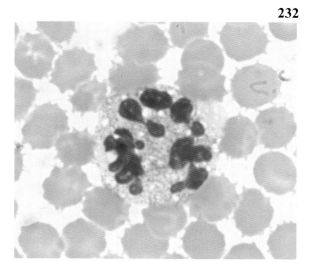

**231** A necrotic white cell in a stored blood sample from a Chinese alligator.

**232** A structure resembling a giant neutrophil from a chimpanzee blood sample which had been in transit for several days.

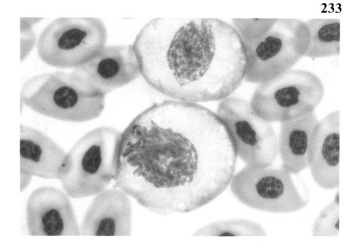

**233** Two cells of unknown origin contaminating a 'blood sample' collected at *post mortem* from a cobra. These are not blood cells.

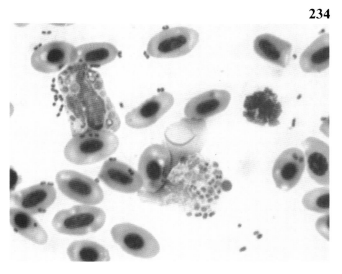

**234** Postal sample from a sulphur crested cockatoo, contaminated with *Escherichia coli*, visible as extracellular basophilic bodies.

**235**

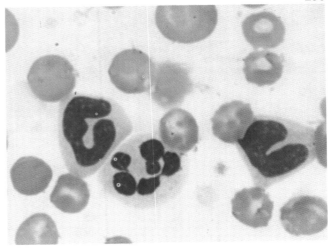

**235** A normal neutrophil and two band neutrophils from a grey wolf with infected skin lesions and marked neutrophilia (neutrophils 62.8 ×10$^9$/l). The finding of neutrophils with reduced nuclear lobulation can be described as a left shift. Except in mammals which show the Pelger-Huët phenomenon and in reptilian species which normally have heterophils with round nuclei, a left shift is a reliable indication of increased cell production, usually in response to infections and other inflammatory conditions. This wolf was also severely anaemic and the red cells show marked anisocytosis, polychromasia, stomatocytosis and microspherocytosis.

**236**

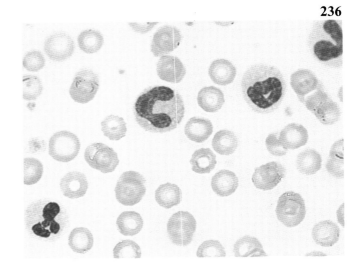

**236** Neutrophilia in a dog with peritonitis. A normal neutrophil and three slightly larger neutrophils showing a left shift are present. The red cells show anisocytosis and hypochromia.

**237**

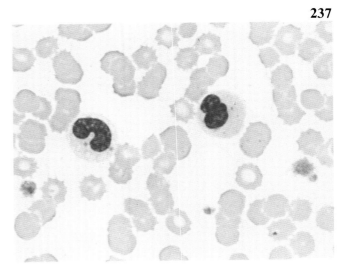

**237** Two band neutrophils from a dog with acute pancreatitis. The cytoplasm of the cell on the right contains toxic granules and that of the cell on the left contains two Döhle bodies. The toxic granules indicate a disturbance in granule formation, resulting in decreased intracellular lysosomal activity. Döhle (Amato) bodies are small blue areas in the cytoplasm consisting of rough endoplasmic reticulum containing RNA. They are thought to represent focal failure of cytoplasmic maturation.

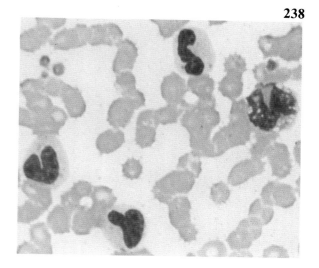

**238** Band neutrophils and a vacuolated monocyte from a dog with bacterial endocarditis. The red cells show increased rouleaux formation.

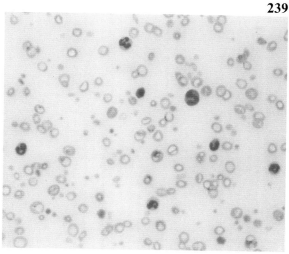

**239** Neutrophilia with a left shift in a dog with a Coombs' positive anaemia (×40). The red cells show marked anisocytosis and hypochromia. One normoblast (erythroblast) is present and the platelet count appears to be increased. Granulocytosis and thrombocytosis are not unusual in regenerative anaemias, caused by generalised marrow stimulation.

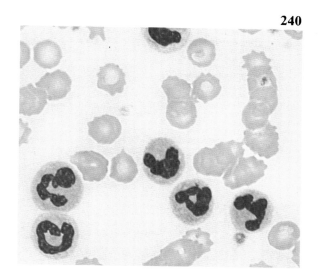

**240** Neutrophilia in a dog with inflammatory disease. The cells do not show a left shift (mature neutrophilia). There is increased red cell rouleaux formation and the platelet count appears to be reduced.

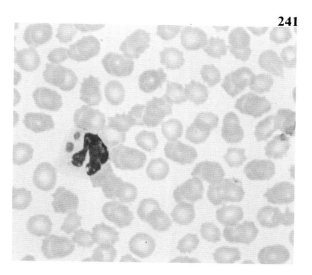

**241** Two eosinophilic inclusion bodies in the cytoplasm of a neutrophil from a dog with distemper. These inclusions, which consist of viral nucleocapsid tubules, can occur also in red cells, lymphocytes and monocytes in cases of canine distemper.

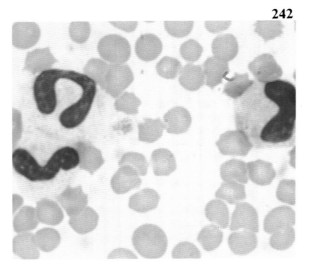

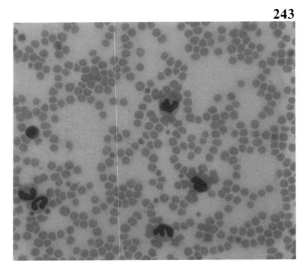

**242** Three band neutrophils from a lion with slight neutrophilia associated with hepatitis (neutrophils 14.4 ×10⁹/l).

**243** Neutrophils showing a left shift from a cat with pyothorax (×40).

**244** Mature neutrophilia in a cat with gastritis (×40, neutrophils 23.7 ×10⁹/l).

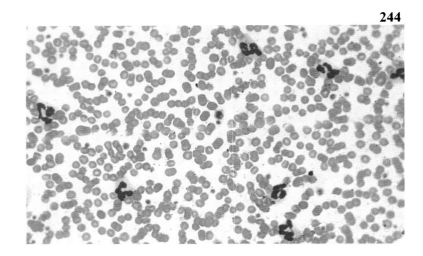

**245** Mature neutrophilia in a cat with a bite abscess (×40).

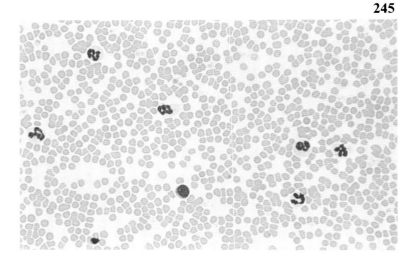

**246** Neutrophilia in a cheetah with acute peritonitis (×40, neutrophils 27.3 ×10⁹/l). Two band neutrophils and four normal neutrophils are shown.

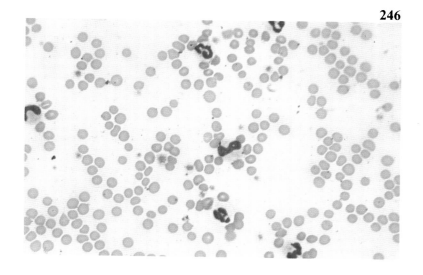

**247** A higher magnification of a normal neutrophil and two neutrophils showing a left shift from the cheetah in **246**.

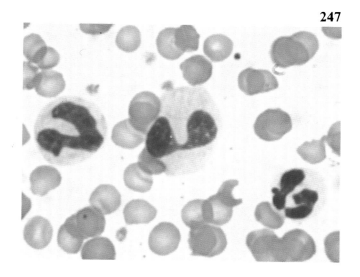

**248** A normal neutrophil and a neutrophil with a ring-form nucleus from the cheetah in **246**. Neutrophils with ring-form nuclei are characteristic of inflammatory disease in carnivores but occur normally in some rodents.

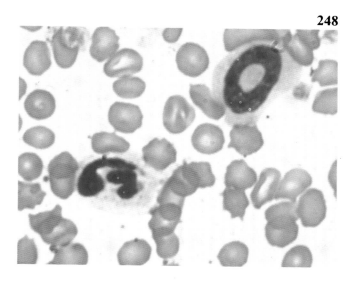

**249** Neutrophilia in a cheetah with acute *Vaccinia variola* (cowpox) infection (neutrophils 44.3 $\times 10^9$/l). The cells have vacuolated cytoplasm and show a marked left shift. One cell with a ring-form nucleus is present.

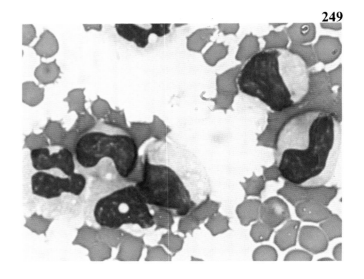

**250** Two neutrophils showing a left shift from a ring-tailed coati with a chronic bacterial infection (neutrophils 17.1 $\times 10^9$/l).

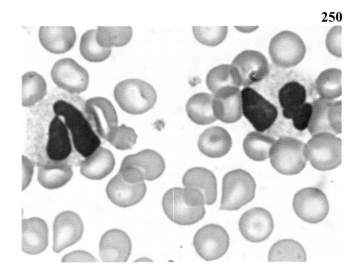

**251** Mature neutrophilia in a crab-eating mongoose with a tooth root abscess ($\times 40$, neutrophils 19.2 $\times 10^9$/l).

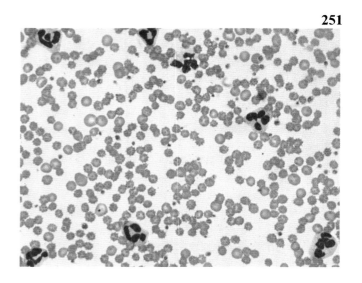

**252** A neutrophil from a chimpanzee with an infected digit. The neutrophil count in this animal was normal (5.3 $\times 10^9$/l) but the presence of infection was suggested by the observation of Döhle bodies and vacuoles in the cells.

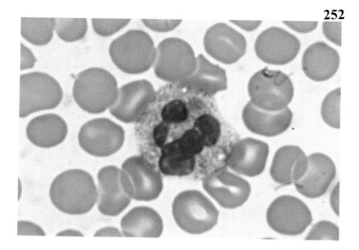

252

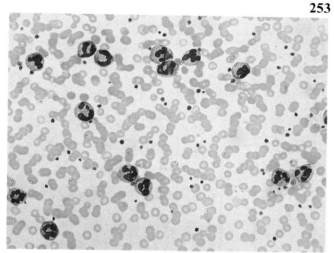

253

**253** Mature neutrophilia in a Barbary ape with tracheitis (×40, neutrophils 33.2 $\times 10^9$/l). This animal also had an abnormally high platelet count.

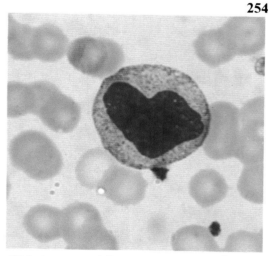

254

**254** A neutrophil metamyelocyte from the ape in **253**.

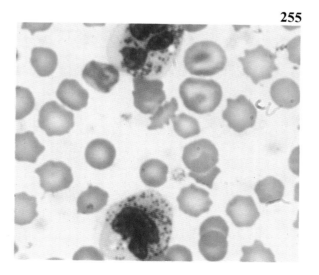

255

**255** A neutrophil showing toxic granulation and vacuolation from a slender loris with a chronic facial abscess (neutrophils 9.4 $\times 10^9$/l).

**256** Neutrophilia in a squirrel monkey with *Yersinia pseudotuberculosis* infection (neutrophils 37.1 ×10⁹/l). Three neutrophils and a monocyte are shown.

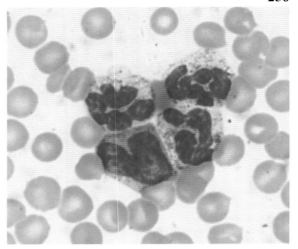

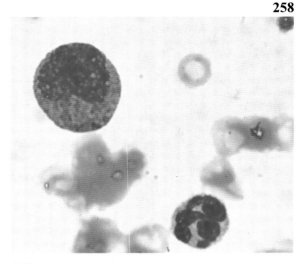

**257** Neutrophilia in an owl monkey with infected, haemorrhagic skin lesions (×40, neutrophils 23.6 ×10⁹/l). Hypochromic anaemia and thrombocytosis are also shown.

**258** A neutrophil myelocyte from the monkey in **257**.

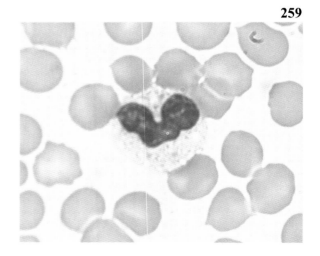

**259** A neutrophil showing a left shift from a Californian sealion with meningitis (neutrophils 16.9 ×10⁹/l). There are several small Döhle bodies in the cytoplasm.

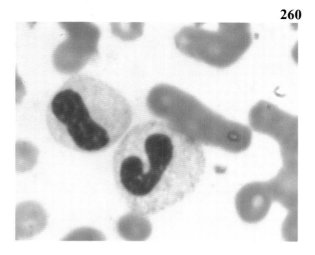

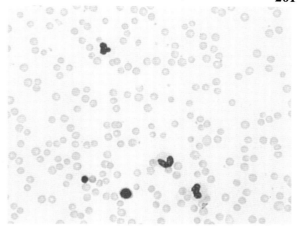

**260** Two band neutrophils from a collared peccary with infected fight wounds (neutrophils 14.5 $\times 10^9$/l). The red cells show increased rouleaux formation.

**261** Band neutrophils from a cow with pyelonephritis, pyuria and haematuria ($\times 40$).

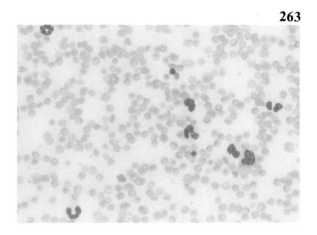

**262** Neutrophilia and monocytosis in a cow with acute mastitis ($\times 40$).

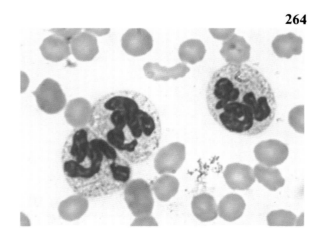

**263** Neutrophilia with a left shift secondary to traumatic reticulitis in a cow, which was anaemic.

**264** Mature neutrophilia in a bighorn sheep with chronic infection (neutrophils 31.9 $\times 10^9$/l). The cells show an increased number of nuclear lobes (right shift).

**265** Two neutrophils showing toxic granulation and cytoplasmic streaming from a nilgai with colitis (neutrophils $20.6 \times 10^9/l$).

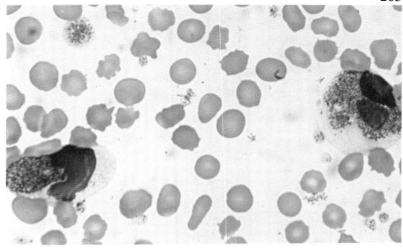

**266** Two band neutrophils with basophilic cytoplasm from a horse with inflammatory disease.

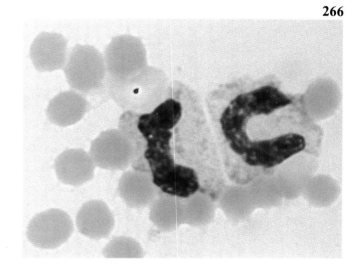

**267** Two overlapping band cells with basophilic cytoplasm from a horse with inflammatory disease.

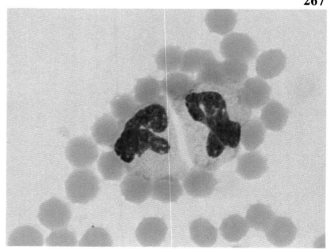

**268** Neutrophilia in a Jamaican hutia with chronic corneal ulceration (neutrophils 19.6 ×10⁹/l). There is no apparent left shift but the cell in the bottom left hand corner of the field contains several Döhle bodies. A monocyte with cytoplasmic vacuoles is also present.

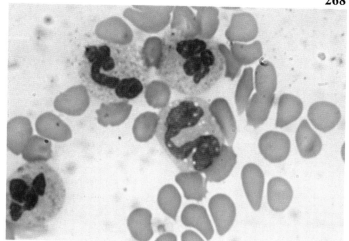
268

**269** Neutrophilia in a casiragua with infected fight wounds (×40, neutrophils 19.8 ×10⁹/l). This animal also had regenerative hypochromic anaemia and thrombocytosis.

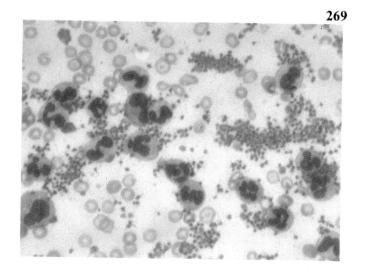
269

**270** A higher magnification of three mature neutrophils and two neutrophils with a left shift from the casiragua in **269**.

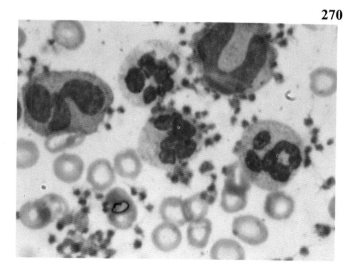
270

**271** Neutrophilia in a plains viscacha with inflammatory disease (×40, neutrophils 36.9 ×10$^9$/l). This animal also had severe hypochromic anaemia and thrombocytosis.

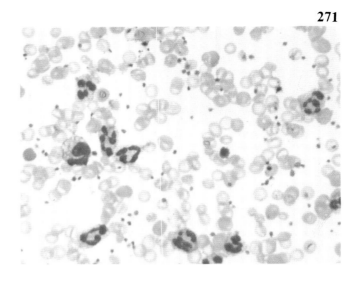

**272** A higher magnification of a mature neutrophil and a band neutrophil with toxic granulation from the viscacha in **271**. The red cells show anisocytosis and hypochromia.

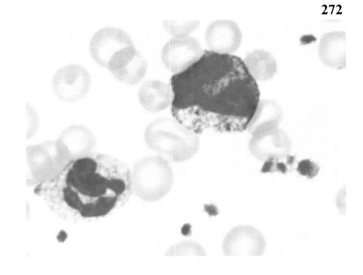

**273** A myeloblast from the viscacha in **271**.

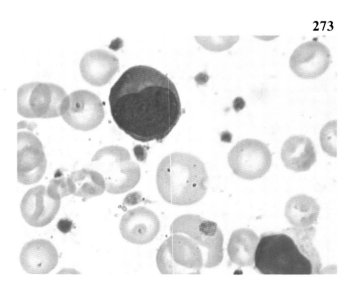

**274** Neutrophils showing a right shift from a large tree shrew with hypervitaminosis A.

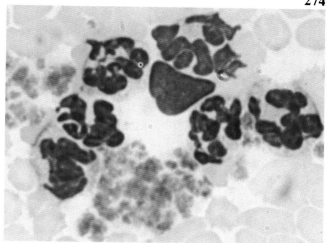

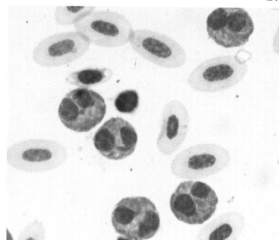

**275** Heterophilia in a blue and gold macaw with chronic respiratory infection (heterophils 41.3 $\times 10^9$/l). This bird was severely anaemic.

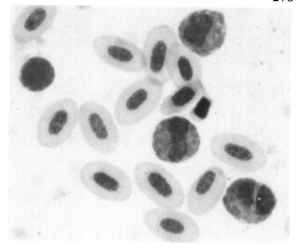

**276** Two heterophils showing a left shift (unlobed nuclei) and a normal heterophil from the macaw in **275**.

**277** Two abnormal heterophils from an Amazon green parrot with an upper respiratory tract infection (heterophils 44.1$\times 10^9$/l). The cells contain irregular eosinophilic granules and an extra complement of round, strongly basophilic granules of varying sizes. These are considered to indicate immaturity or toxicity.

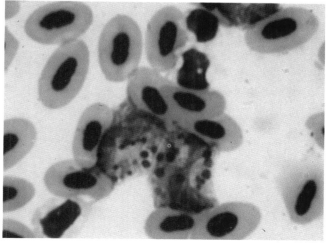

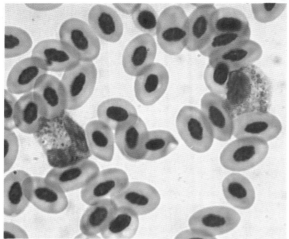

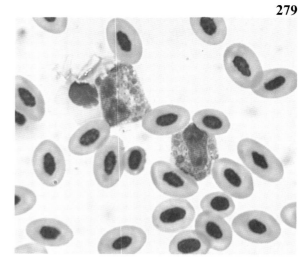

**278** Toxic heterophil from a Buffon's macaw with chronic viral hepatitis and peritonitis (heterophils $8.5 \times 10^9$/l). Both heterophils have irregular cytoplasmic granules and one has an unlobed nucleus.

**279** Two abnormal heterophils from the macaw in **278**. Some of the cytoplasmic granules are round and comparatively large and have a basophilic tinge.

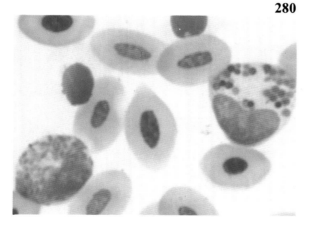

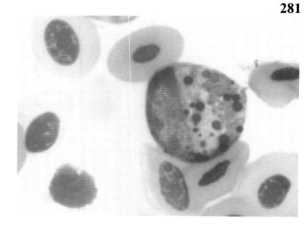

**280** Abnormal heterophils from an ostrich suffering from anorexia and weight loss (heterophils $3.7 \times 10^9$/l). The cause of the illness was not known but the appearance of the heterophils in the absence of an increased count suggested a degenerative white cell response to an infectious condition.

**281** A heterophil myelocyte from the ostrich in **280**.

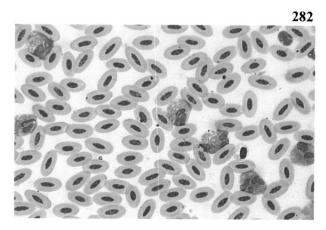

**282** Heterophilia in a rosy flamingo with cellulitis ($\times 40$, heterophils $17.6 \times 10^9$/l).

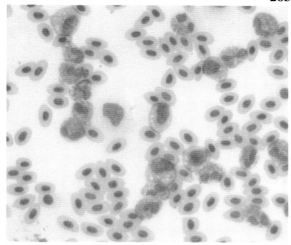

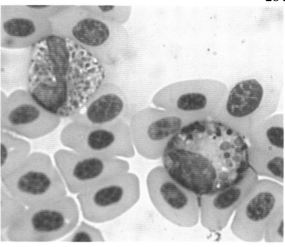

**283** Heterophilia and monocytosis in a domestic fowl with *Mycobacterium avium* infection (×40, heterophils 134.1 ×10$^9$/l).

**284** An immature heterophil with an unlobed nucleus, a reduced number of eosinophilic granules and a number of round basophilic granules from the bird in **283**. A normal heterophil is also present.

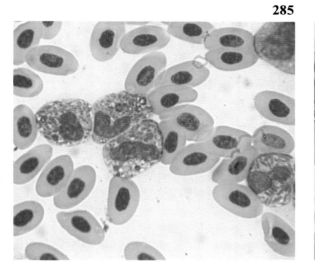

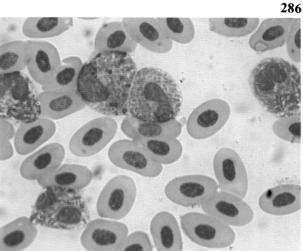

**285, 286** Heterophils from the bird in **283** showing varying degrees of nuclear and granule abnormalities.

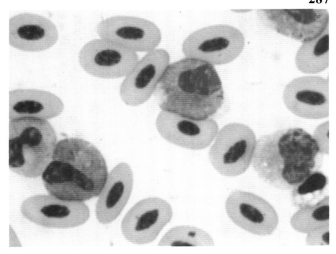

**287** Heterophils showing a left shift and a normal eosinophil (left) from a hooded crane with *Mycobacterium avium* infection (heterophils 30.1 $\times 10^9$/l).

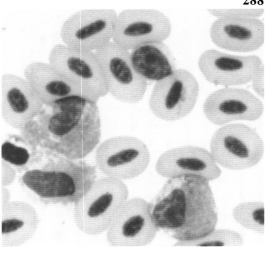

**288** Two more band heterophils, a band eosinophil, a normal lymphocyte and a normal thrombocyte from the crane in **287**.

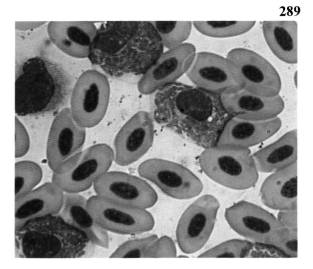

**289** Three heterophils with unlobed nuclei from a sarus crane with *Mycobacterium avium* infection (heterophils 33.6 $\times 10^9$/l). An unidentified disintegrating mononuclear cell is also present.

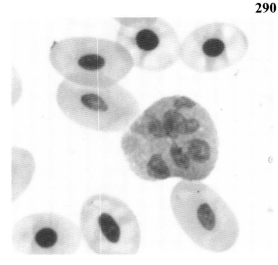

**290** A giant heterophil with a hypersegmented nucleus from a blackfooted penguin with aspergillosis. The bird had heterophilia (20.6 $\times 10^9$/l), monocytosis and normochromic anaemia.

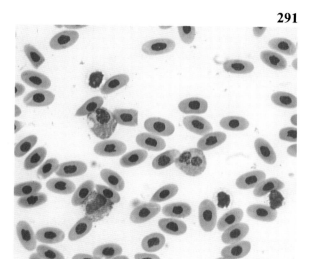

**291** Heterophilia with a left shift in a common iguana with a fractured hind limb (×40, heterophils 12.3 ×10$^9$/l). The heterophils of this species normally have lobed nuclei.

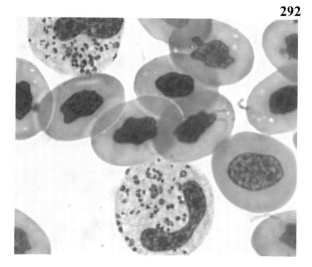

**292** Heterophils with band-form nuclei and abnormal (toxic?) cytoplasmic granules from a blue-tongued skink with multiple abscesses (heterophils 3.1 ×10$^9$/l). The heterophils of skinks normally have distinctively bilobed nuclei. Heterophilia is relatively uncommon in reptiles with inflammatory diseases and the presence of heterophils with morphological abnormalities is often the most useful indicator of infection in these animals.

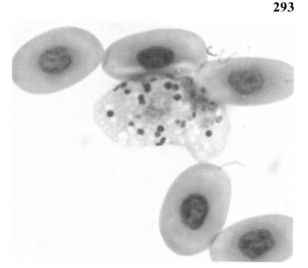

**293, 294** Abnormal heterophils from a LeSueur's water dragon with osteomyelitis (heterophils 1.1 ×10$^9$/l). In water dragons the heterophil nucleus is normally round.

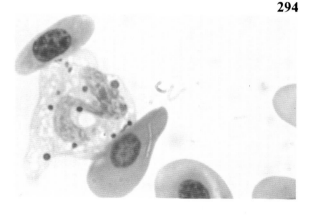

**295** Abnormal heterophils from a green water dragon with blepharitis (heterophils 9.2 ×10$^9$/l). The nuclei are slightly lobed with clumping of the chromatin. The cytoplasm is grey and the granules are irregular in shape and reduced in number. One of the cells shows cytoplasmic vacuolation.

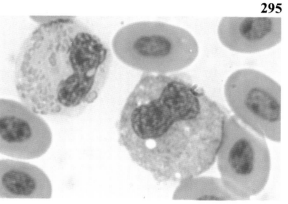

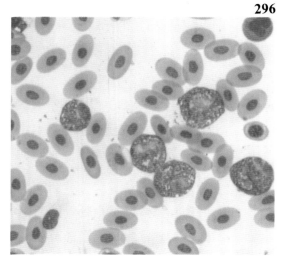

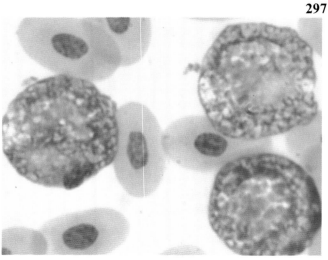

**296** Heterophilia in an Eastern fox snake with severe spreading necrosis of the tail (heterophils 23.6 $\times 10^9$/l). This snake also had marked azurophilia.

**297** A higher magnification of three abnormal heterophils from the snake in **296**. The cells are macrocytic and the unlobed nuclei have not taken up the stain.

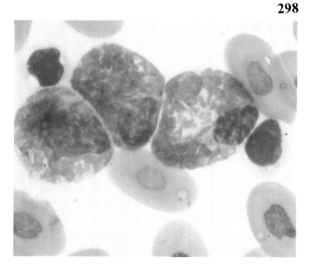

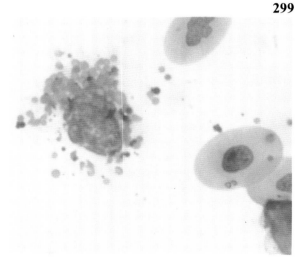

**298** Three heterophils from a carpet python with cellulitis, multiple abscesses and muscle necrosis (heterophils 3.4 $\times 10^9$/l). The cytoplasmic granules are irregular in shape and there is variation in stain uptake. This snake also had azurophilia.

**299** A ruptured heterophil from the snake in **298**, revealing the presence of abnormal granules.

**300, 301** Abnormal heterophils from a Montpelier snake with ascites and cloacal haemorrhage. This snake had a low heterophil count (heterophils $0.3 \times 10^9/l$), anaemia and azurophilia. The heterophils show abnormal nuclear lobulation (the heterophils of snakes normally have round nuclei), grey cytoplasm and toxic granulation.

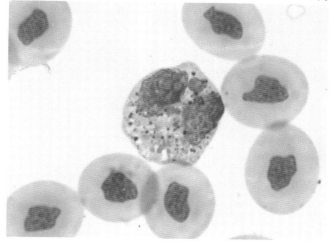

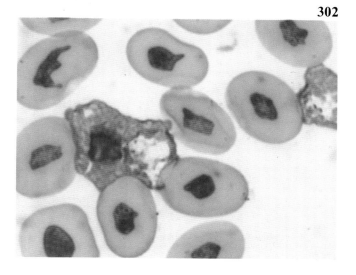

**302** Abnormal heterophils from a hawksbill turtle with suspected liver failure (heterophils $3.6 \times 10^9/l$). The nuclei of the red cells are distorted.

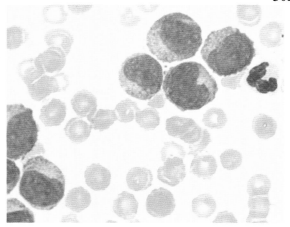

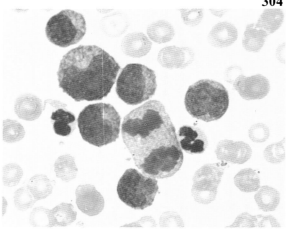

**303** Promyelocytes and a normal neutrophil from a dog with chronic myeloid (granulocytic) leukaemia. The red cells show increased rouleaux formation and platelets are absent.

**304** Five myeloblasts, a promyelocyte, two normal neutrophils and a mitotic figure from the dog in **303**.

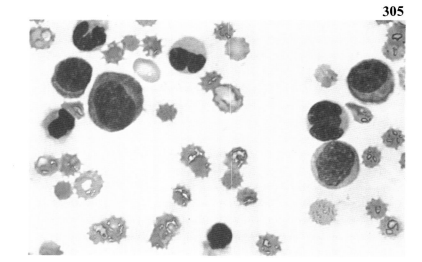

**305** Promyelocytes and band neutrophils in a dog with chronic myeloid leukaemia. The red cells show crenation and anisocytosis and platelets are absent.

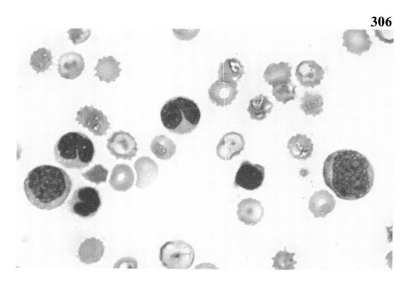

**306** Myeloblasts and band neutrophils from the dog in **305**.

**307** Chronic myeloid leukaemia in a cat (×40). This animal was strongly FeLV-positive.

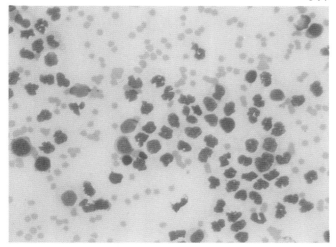

**308** Chronic myeloid leukaemia in a cat.

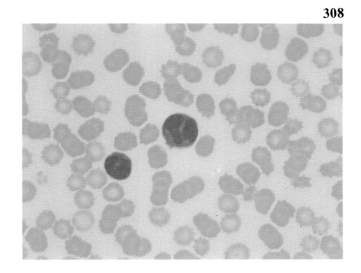

**309** Bone marrow preparation from the cat in **308** with chronic myeloid leukaemia.

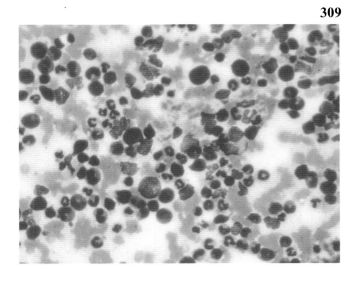

**310** Chronic myeloid leukaemia in transition to acute myeloid leukaemia in a dog (×40). Many myeloblasts and five normal neutrophils are present. There are also several disintegrating cells.

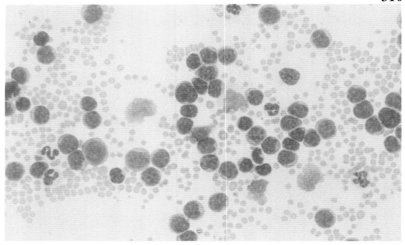

**311** Cells from the dog in **310** at higher magnification.

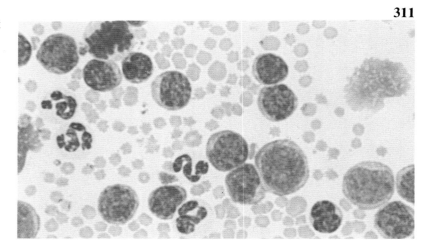

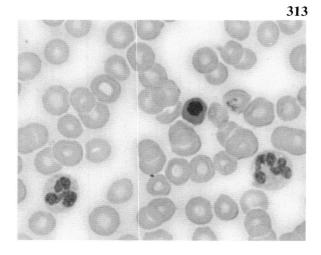

**312** A pleiomorphic population of myeloblasts in the peripheral blood of a dog with acute myeloid leukaemia.

**313** A normoblast (erythroblast) and abnormally segmented neutrophils in the blood of a dog with myeloid dysplasia.

**314** Two normal neutrophils and an abnormal metamyelocyte(?) in a dog with a testicular tumour (neutrophils 41.7×10⁹/l).

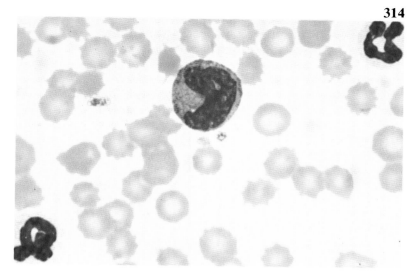

**315** Eosinophilia in a cheetah (×40, eosinophils 4.1 ×10⁹/l). One normal neutrophil is present.

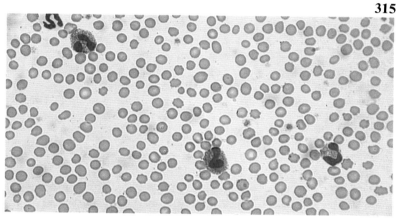

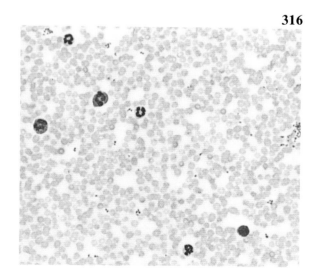

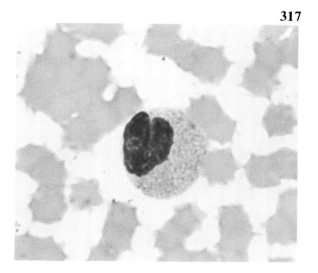

**316** Eosinophilia in a cat with bronchial asthma (×40). The eosinophil nuclei are multilobed.

**317** A higher magnification of an eosinophil from the cat in **316**. The cytoplasm appears to contain Döhle bodies.

103

**318** Eosinophilia in a cat with clinically significant *Aleurostrongylus abstrusus* infestation.

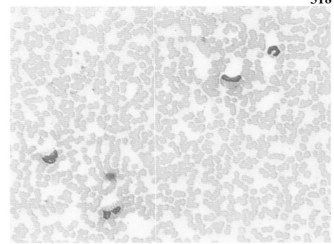

**318**

**319** An eosinophil from a dog with *Filaroides osleri* parasites.

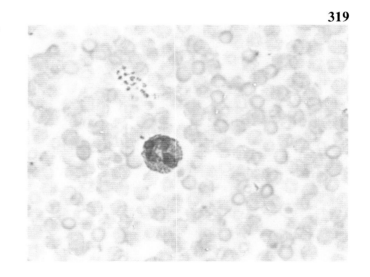

**319**

**320** Eosinophilia and basophilia in a sheep with a heavy *Haemonchus contortus* burden. There is also a normal neutrophil in the field.

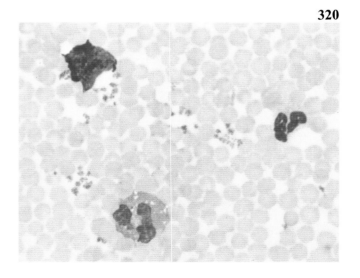

**320**

**321** A vacuolated eosinophil from a ring-tailed coati with haemolytic anaemia of unknown aetiology (eosinophils 0.01 $\times 10^9$/l).

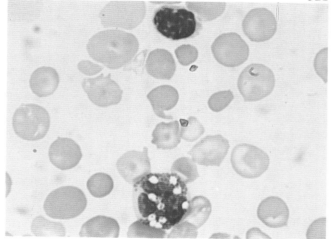

**322** Myeloid hyperplasia and vacuolated eosinophil precursors in the bone marrow of the coati in **321**.

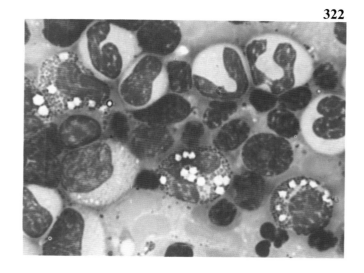

**323** Eosinophilia in a lappet-faced vulture (eosinophils 1.2 $\times 10^9$/l). This bird was clinically normal but was probably suffering from a sub-clinical parasite infestation.

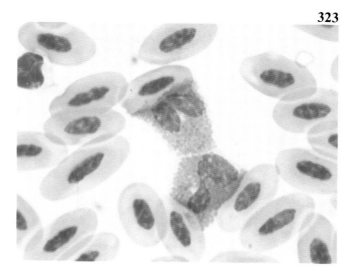

**324** Mast cells in the peripheral blood of a cat with a solid mast cell tumour (mast cells $10.1 \times 10^9$/l). In cats and dogs, mast cells in the peripheral blood can be distinguished from basophils by their unlobed nuclei and the very large number of basophilic granules. There were very few of these cells in the bone marrow of this cat but many in the spleen and liver.

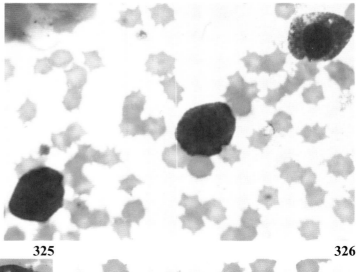

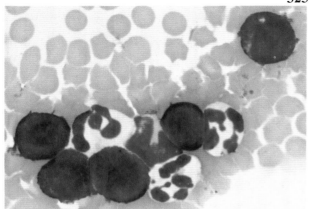

**325** Mast cells in the 'tail' of a blood film from the cat in **324**.

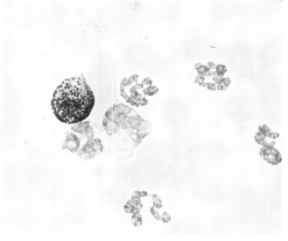

**326** A vacuolated mast cell from the cat in **324**.

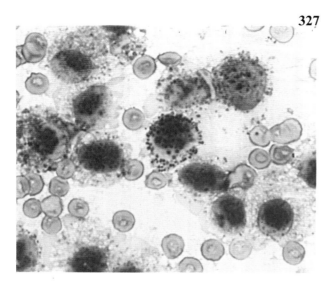

**327** Mast cells in a buffy coat preparation from a dog with a solid mast cell tumour.

**328** A mast cell and several unstained neutrophils in the blood of a dog with a solid mast cell tumour (toluidine blue stain).

# Part 3
# Normal and Abnormal Lymphocytes, Monocytes and Azurophils

## Lymphocytes

Typical lymphocytes are regular, round cells with round, central or slightly excentric, round nuclei and a varying amount of clear, pale blue cytoplasm. They are present in the blood of all mammals, birds and reptiles. In some species, the cytoplasm of a proportion of the cells contains a few azurophilic or basophilic granules. In blood films made from avian or reptilian blood, the lymphocytes often appear to be deformed by close juxtaposition of red cells. In birds and particularly in reptiles, it can be difficult to distinguish between lymphocytes and thrombocytes; this is usually easier in samples in which partial activation of the thrombocytes has occurred. Some practice is needed to avoid the misidentification of disrupted avian and reptilian red cells as lymphocytes.

Lymphocytes are concerned with immunological reactions and, in mammals and birds, can be divided into two main groups with different functions and membrane properties. These are the B lymphocytes which produce immunoglobulins and T lymphocytes which are responsible for cell mediated immunity. B and T lymphocytes cannot be differentiated without the use of specialised techniques which are beyond the scope of this Atlas.

Lymphopoiesis takes place in the spleen and thymus and, additionally, in the tonsillar glands of reptiles, the bursa of Fabricius in birds and the lymph nodes, Peyer's patches and to some extent in the bone marrow in mammals. Immature lymphocytes are distinguished from mature forms by their larger size, increased cytoplasmic basophilia and by the presence of nucleoli. In juvenile animals of many species, the lymphocyte is the predominant white cell in the bloodstream and in some species this situation persists throughout life. A pathological increase in lymphocytes occurs in some virus infections and lymphoproliferative disorders. Lymphopenia can be associated with stress.

## Monocytes

Monocytes are usually larger than lymphocytes and can be distinguished by the presence of a relatively pale staining, kidney-shaped nucleus and abundant, slightly opaque, blue-grey cytoplasm which may appear faintly granular. They are found in the blood of all mammals and birds and probably occur in lower numbers in all reptiles. In most species, monocytes are relatively uncommon but in elephants, cells with distinctly bilobed nuclei and blue-grey cytoplasm, which have the cytochemical characteristics of monocytes, occur in large numbers.

Monocytes are derived from promonocytes in the bone marrow and circulate in the bloodstream before entering the tissues as mature macrophages. Their main functions depend upon their phagocytic activity against invading organisms, necrotic cells and cell debris and on their ability to concentrate antibody for presentation to the lymphocytes. Monocytosis occurs in some bacterial infections including tuberculosis and brucellosis, some protozoal, viral and fungal infections, malignant conditions and collagen diseases and also during recovery from acute infections. In many mammalian species, the monocyte count is higher in juveniles than in adults.

## Azurophils

Azurophils occur only in the blood of reptiles where they are found in low numbers in normal lizards, crocodilians and chelonians and in higher numbers in snakes. They are mononuclear cells, the shape of which can vary from round, lymphocyte-like cells to larger cells which have a monocytoid appearance. These different forms may represent stages in cell maturation. An outstanding feature of azurophils is the metachromic reaction of their cytoplasm with Romanowsky stains. This makes the cell relatively easy to recognise in routine blood films.

Information is lacking about the origin and function of azurophils and these cells have been variously considered as allied to the granulocyte or monocyte series. There is little doubt that they play some part in the inflammatory response, particularly in snakes, and azurophilia and/or 'toxic' changes in cell morphology are usually indicative of infection.

**329-357** *Normal variations in lymphocyte morphology.*

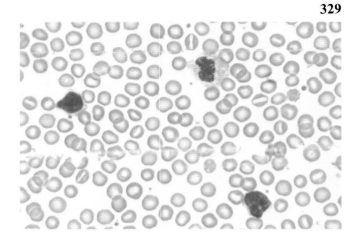

**329** Two normal lymphocytes and a monocyte from a juvenile anubis baboon (×40).

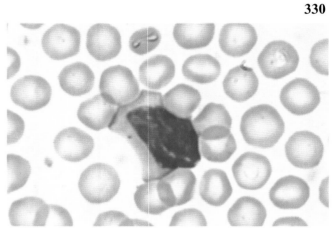

**330** A higher magnification of a normal large lymphocyte from the baboon in **329**. The cell is deformed by the surrounding red cells.

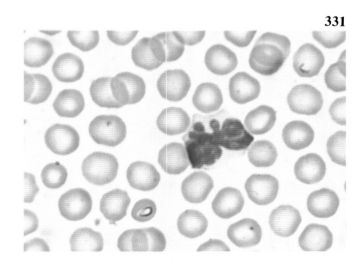

**331** An atypical lymphocyte from the baboon in **329**.

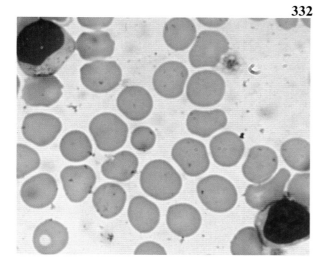

**332** Two normal lymphocytes from a healthy juvenile white-headed saki monkey.

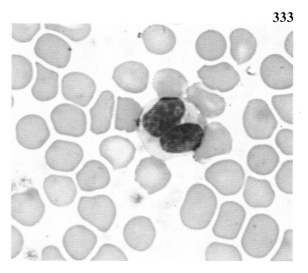

**333** A binucleated lymphocyte from the monkey in **332**. These occur occasionally in the blood of normal primates.

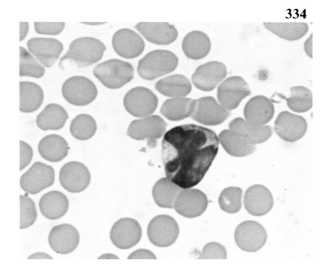

**334** An atypical lymphocyte from a healthy adult brown capuchin monkey.

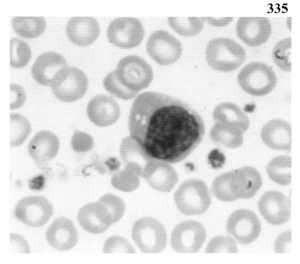

**335** A lymphocyte with small cytoplasmic vacuoles from a healthy orang utan.

**336** Two normal lymphocytes and a normal neutrophil from an owl monkey. The cytoplasm of one of the lymphocytes contains distinctive basophilic granules at the periphery.

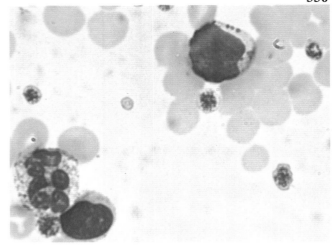

**337** Two normal lymphocytes from a red-necked wallaby. In this species, the nuclear chromatin typically forms dark-staining blocks and the amount of cytoplasm present is often small.

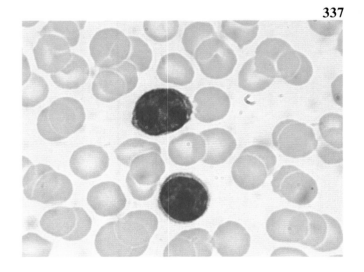

**338** A large lymphocyte from a healthy masked palm civet.

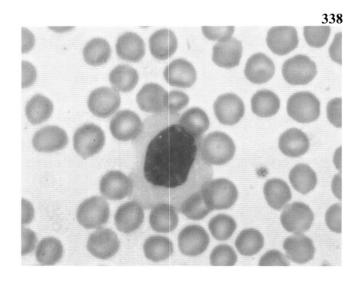

**339** A lymphocyte with azurophilic cytoplasmic granules from a healthy rat.

**339**

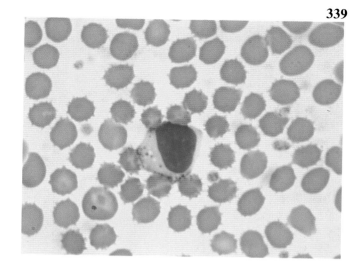

**340** A lymphocyte containing a Kurloff body from a guinea pig. Kurloff bodies are single, large cytoplasmic inclusions which occur under normal conditions in a small proportion of the lymphocytes of this species. In the cell shown, the Kurloff body is below the nucleus.

**340**

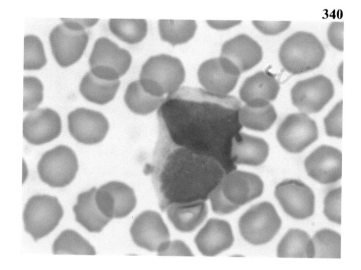

**341** A lymphocyte containing a Kurloff body from a capybara, the only species other than guinea pigs in which these inclusions have been found. The Kurloff body shows signs of disintegration.

**341**

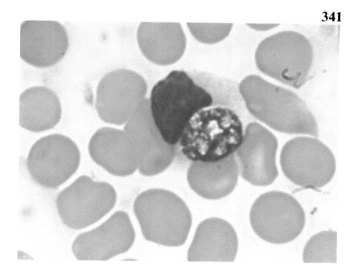

**342** Two lymphocytes from a healthy Arabian camel.

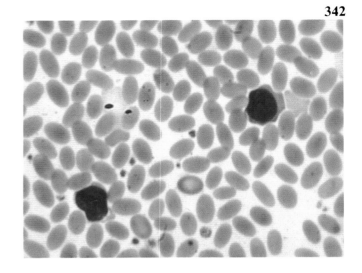

**343** Two normal lymphocytes from a moorhen. These show the typical appearance of avian lymphocytes, which often look deformed in stained blood films. Two thrombocytes with smaller, more condensed nuclei are also present.

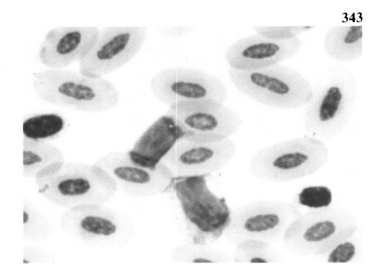

**344** A lymphocyte and a normal thrombocyte from a Javan fish owl.

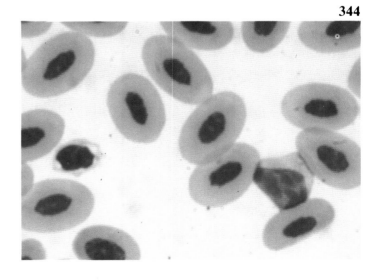

**345** A normal lymphocyte and two thrombocytes from a hill mynah.

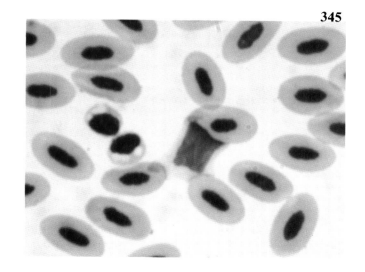

**346** A normal lymphocyte, an aggregate of four thrombocytes showing various stages of activation, two nuclei from red cells which have lost their cytoplasm, a polychromatic erythroblast and a ruptured red cell from a healthy ostrich.

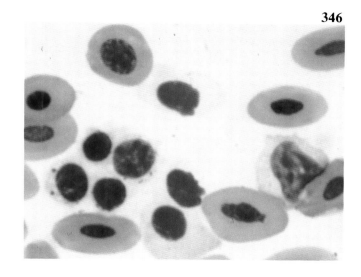

**347** A lymphocyte, a thrombocyte (with cytoplasmic vacuoles) and several polychromatic red cells from a budgerigar.

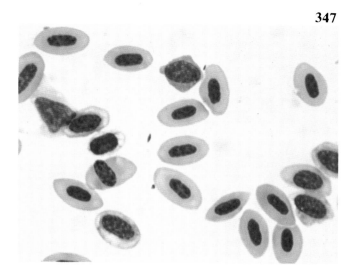

**348** A normal lymphocyte from a rosy flamingo.

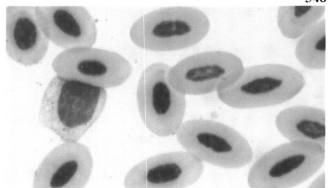

**349** Two lymphocytes and a heterophil from a hooded crane with *Mycobacterium avium* infection. Several large basophilic granules are present in the cytoplasm of the lymphocytes; these also occur in lymphocytes from healthy cranes. The heterophil has a band nucleus.

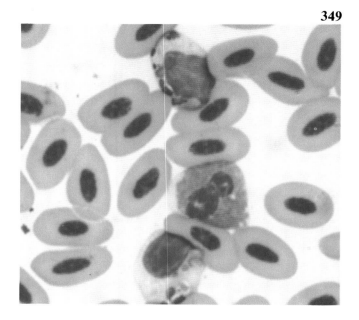

**350** A small lymphocyte with cytoplasmic granules and a monocyte from a sarus crane.

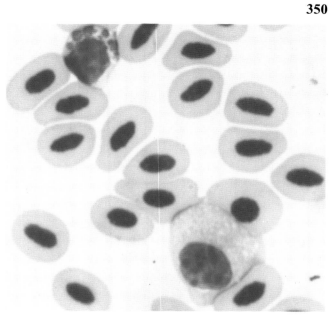

**351** A normal lymphocyte (top) and two thrombocytes from a healthy taipan snake. Reptilian lymphocytes usually appear less deformable than those of birds. The thrombocytes can be distinguished by their irregular, vacuolated cytoplasm.

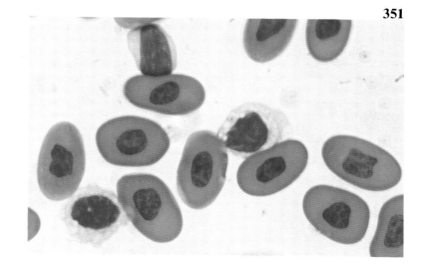

351

**352** Four lymphocytes and a thrombocyte from the snake in **351**. Two of the lymphocytes have indented nuclei and one shows an irregularity of the cytoplasmic membrane.

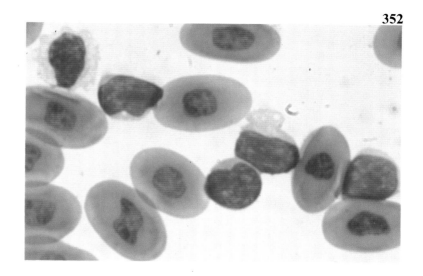

352

**353** A lymphocyte with heavy cytoplasmic granulation and a normal thrombocyte from a healthy reticulated python.

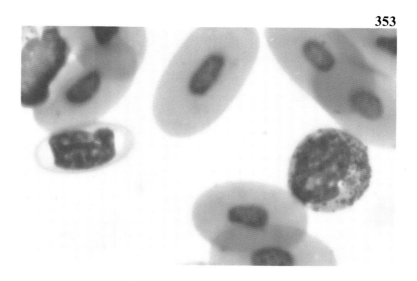

353

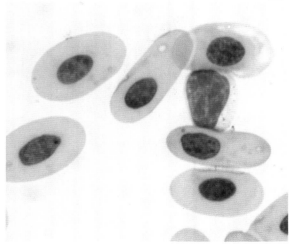

**354** A lymphocyte from a healthy spur-thighed tortoise.

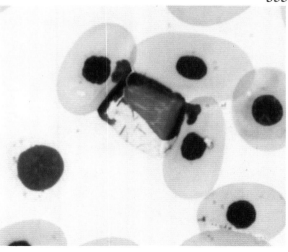

**355** A lymphocyte with rod-shaped cytoplasmic granules from a healthy red-eared terrapin.

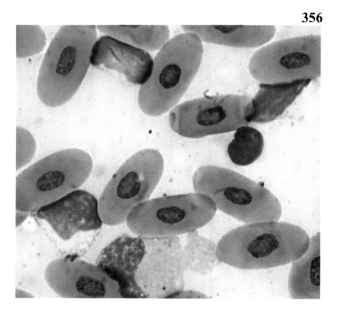

**356** Three lymphocytes, a thrombocyte and a monocyte from a healthy rhinoceros iguana. The cytoplasm of two of the lymphocytes contains faint eosinophilic granules. The monocyte shows signs of disintegration.

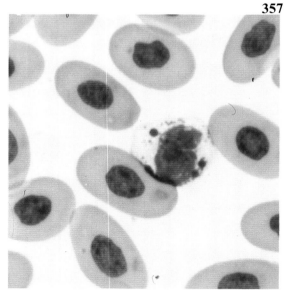

**357** A lymphocyte with large basophilic cytoplasmic granules from a healthy LeSueur's water dragon.

**358-388** *Abnormalities in the lymphocytes associated with disease.*

**358**

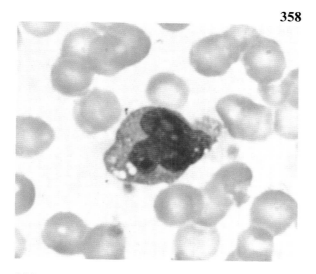

**359**

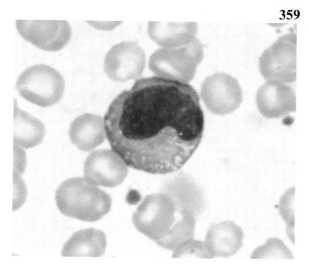

**358** An abnormal lymphocyte from a cynomol-gus (crab-eating) macaque with chronic peritoni-tis (lymphocytes $4.0 \times 10^9$/l). The cell has an irregularly shaped nucleus and the cytoplasm shows vacuolation.

**359** An abnormal lymphocyte from the macaque in **358**.

**360**

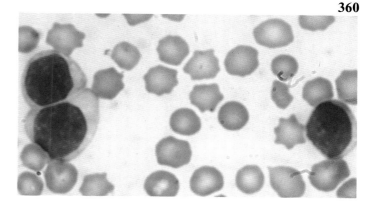

**360** Three normal lymphocytes from a slender loris with lymphocytosis (lymphocytes $13.5 \times 10^9$/l). The cells show a tendency to aggregate. This animal had a facial abscess but the cause of the lymphocytosis was not known.

**361**

**361** A lymphocyte with numerous cytoplasmic granules from the loris in **360**.

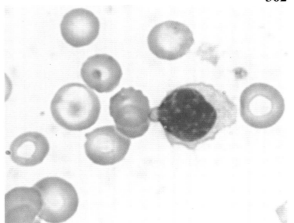

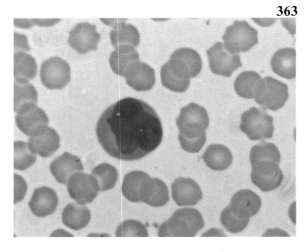

**362** A lymphocyte with an irregular cytoplasmic membrane from a ring-tailed coati with auto-immune haemolytic anaemia.

**363** An active lymphocyte (virocyte, immunoblast) from a masked palm civet with a respiratory infection (lymphocytes 5.3 $\times 10^9$/l). The cell has strongly basophilic cytoplasm.

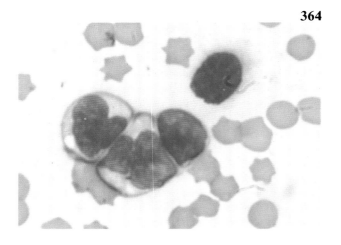

**364** Abnormal lymphocytes from a cat with lymphoma. This animal had lymphopenia (lymphocytes 0.4 $\times 10^9$/l) and the cells show a tendency to aggregate together. The two larger cells with nuclear cleavage are lymphoma cells.

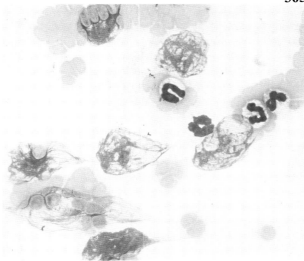

**365** Three normal neutrophils and many basket cells, presumed to be disintegrating lymphocytes, in the 'tail' of a blood film from a dog with lymphoma (lymphocytes 4.5 $\times 10^9$/l).

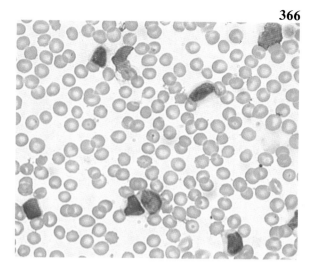

**366**

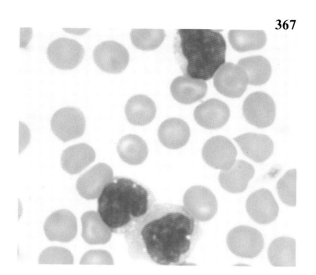

**367**

**366** Lymphocytosis in a dog with untreated lymphocytic lymphoma (×40, lymphocytes 60.8 ×10$^9$/l). Thrombocytopenia is also evident.

**367** A higher magnification of lymphocytes from the dog in **366**. The cells show nuclear cleavage and cytoplasmic vacuolation typical of lymphoma cells and a tendency to aggregate together.

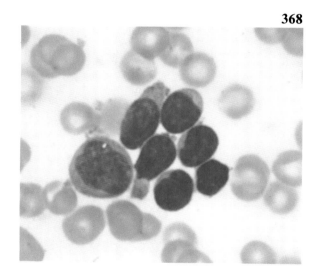

**368**

**368** A group of six abnormal lymphocytes, probably lymphoblasts, from the dog in **366**.

**369** A blood film from the dog in **366** after treatment with steroids (×40, lymphocytes 6.1 ×10$^9$/l). Two lymphocytes and two disintegrating white cells (basket cells) are shown. Thrombocytopenia is still evident from the lack of platelets on the film and the dog died a few days later from acute haemorrhage.

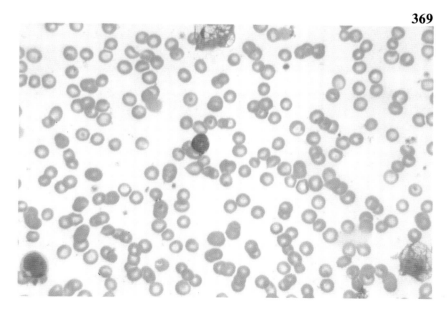

**369**

**370** Lymphoblastic overflow in the blood of a cat with multicentric lymphosarcoma.

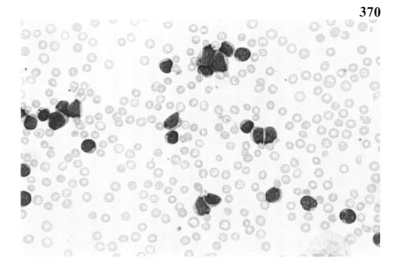

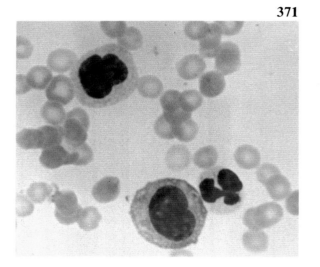

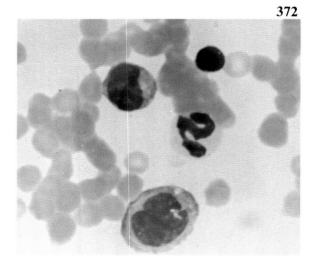

**371, 372** Lymphosarcoma in a horse.

**373** One normal lymphocyte and many lymphoblasts from a dog with lymphoblastic leukaemia. The red cells show hypochromia, crenation, and ovalocytosis. The dog also had thrombocytopenia.

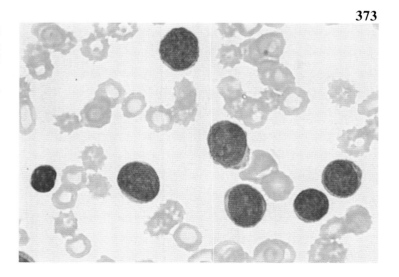

**374-379** *Lymphoid leukaemia in cats.*

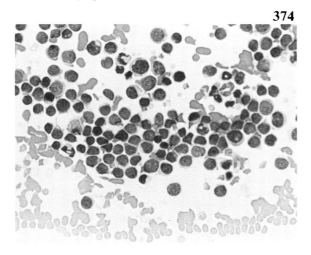

374

374 General view of a blood film from a case of unclassified lymphoid leukaemia.

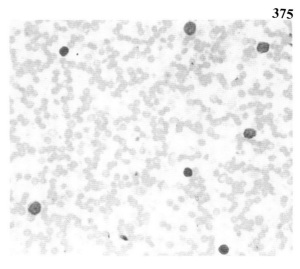

375

375 Chronic lymphocytic leukaemia (×40). The lymphocyte count is increased but the cell morphology is unremarkable.

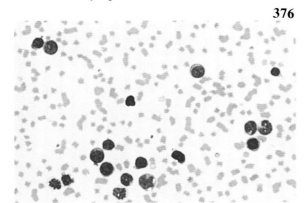

376

376 Lymphocytosis with some cells showing abnormal morphology in a case of chronic lymphocytic leukaemia (×40).

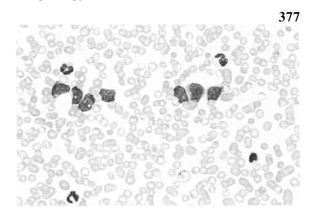

377

377 Chronic lymphocytic leukaemia (×40).

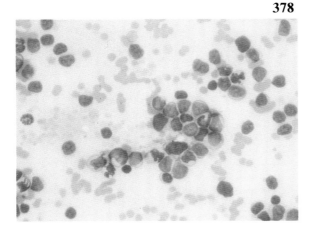

378

378 Lymphoblasts in a case of acute lymphoblastic leukaemia (×40).

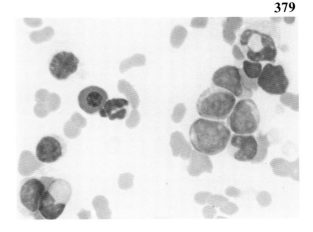

379

379 A higher magnification of lymphoblasts in the cat in 378.

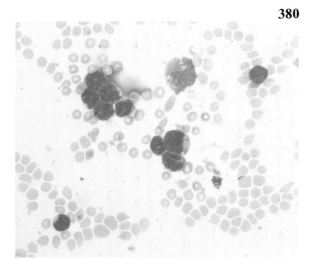

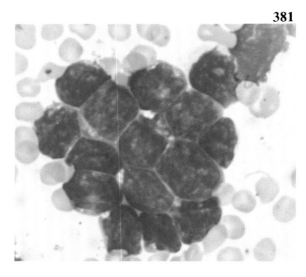

**380** Acute lymphoblastic leukaemia in a mouse lemur (×40, lymphocytes 138.9 ×10$^9$/l). The lymphoblasts show a marked tendency to aggregate. This animal also had severe, regenerative normocytic anaemia and thrombocytopenia.

**381** A higher magnification of an aggregate of lymphoblasts from the lemur in **380**.

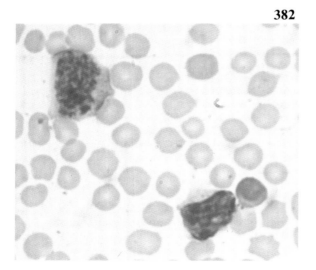

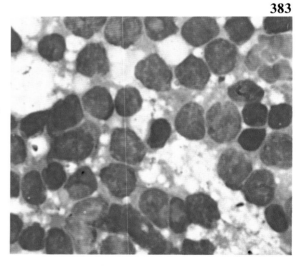

**382** Two abnormal lymphocytes from the lemur in **380**. The red cells show polychromasia.

**383** A bone marrow sample from the lemur in **380**, obtained immediately after death, showing massive lymphoblast infiltration.

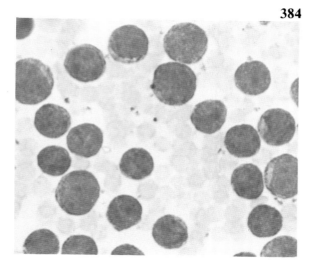

**384** Lymphoid leukaemia in a sheep.

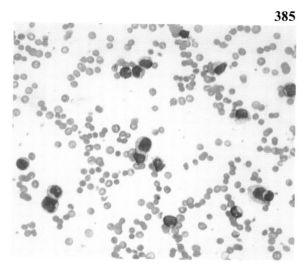

**385** Lymphocytic leukaemia in a rat (×25, lymphocytes 49.2 ×10$^9$/l). The lymphocytes have irregular nuclei with a loose chromatin pattern and the cytoplasm of many is vacuolated and contains prominent basophilic granules. This animal also had neutropenia, thrombocytopenia and severe regenerative macrocytic anaemia.

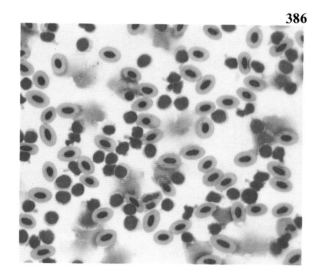

**386** Lymphocytosis in a mallard with a lymphoid leucosis (lymphocytes 127.0 ×10$^9$/l). The cells show some tendency to aggregate.

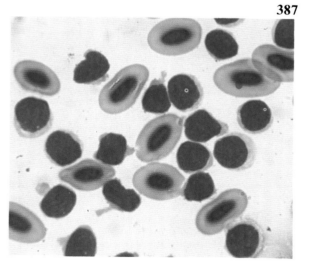

**387** Lymphoblasts from the duck in **386**, some of which show irregularities of the cytoplasmic membrane.

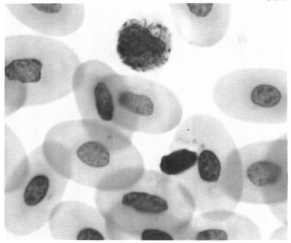

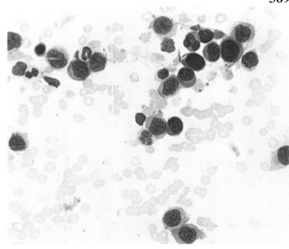

**388** A lymphocyte(?) containing phagocytised material from an Indian python with dermatitis (lymphocytes $0.5 \times 10^9/l$).

**389** Plasma cells in the bone marrow of a case of myeloma in a dog.

**390–398** *Normal monocyte morphology.*

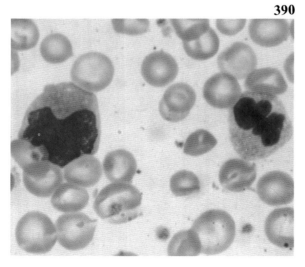

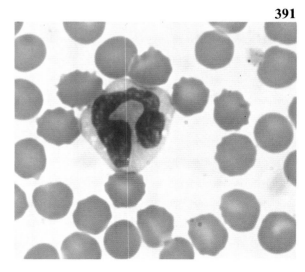

**390** A typical monocyte and a neutrophil from a healthy cotton-top tamarin.

**391** A typical monocyte from a healthy dog.

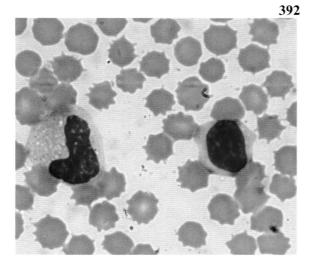

**392** A normal monocyte (left) and lymphocyte from a healthy gaur. The red cells are crenated.

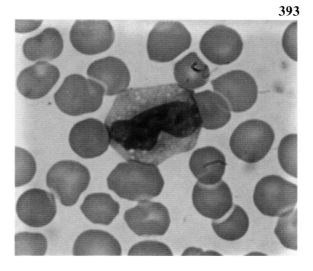

**393** A monocyte from a healthy capybara.

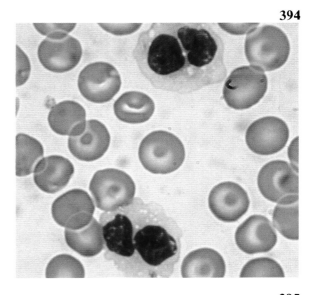

**394** Two normal bilobed mononuclear cells from a healthy Indian elephant. Cells of this type are found in both Indian and African elephants and are classified as monocytes on the basis of their cytochemical staining reactions. The number of these cells present in healthy animals is significantly greater than the number of monocytes found in other mammals and is increased in juveniles and in individuals with inflammatory disease.

**395** A trilobed monocyte from the elephant in **394**.

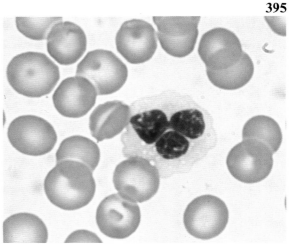

**396** A monocyte from a healthy rosy flamingo.

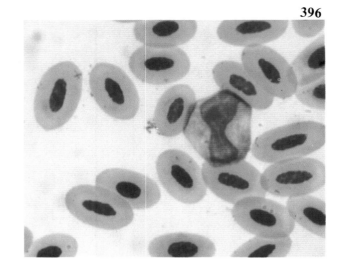
396

**397** A monocyte with cytoplasmic vacuoles from a healthy ostrich.

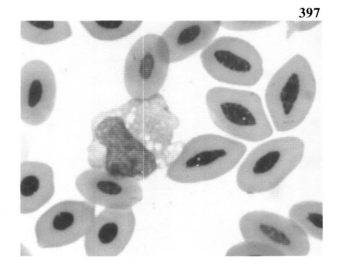
397

**398** A monocyte from a healthy common iguana.

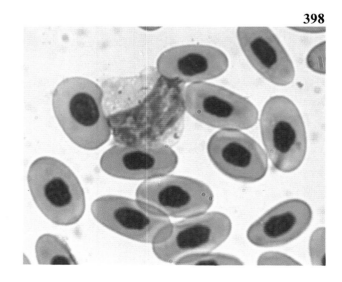
398

**399-418** *Abnormal monocytes.*

**399** A monocyte with an irregular nucleus and cytoplasmic vacuolation from a slender loris with a facial abscess. This animal had a high lymphocyte count and a slight monocytosis (monocytes $0.9 \times 10^9/l$). A neutrophil with toxic granulation is also present.

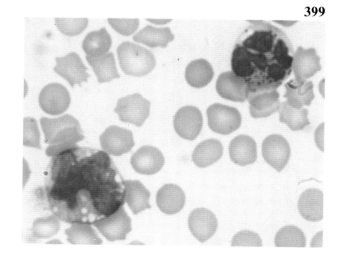

**400** Two monocytes with cytoplasmic vacuoles from a ruffed lemur with chronic respiratory disease (monocytes $1.0 \times 10^9/l$).

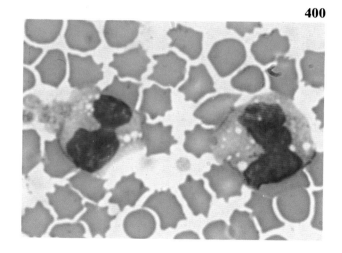

**401** Two abnormal monocytes from a red-bellied tamarin with an infected and necrotic tail lesion (monocytes $0.9 \times 10^9/l$). One of the monocytes shows extreme nuclear malformation and the nuclei of both contain small vacuoles.

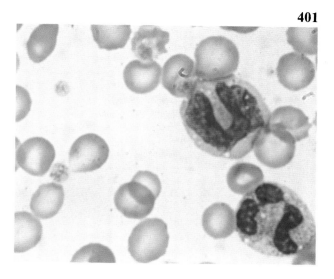

**402** Two abnormal monocytes with cytoplasmic vacuoles from a long-haired spider monkey with *Yersinia pseudotuberculosis* infection (monocytes $1.3 \times 10^9/l$).

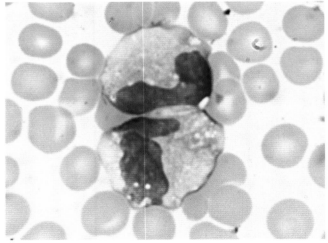

**403** An abnormal monocyte with vacuolated cytoplasm and increased nuclear cleavage from a cynomolgus macaque with haemorrhagic anaemia (monocytes $0.7 \times 10^9/l$).

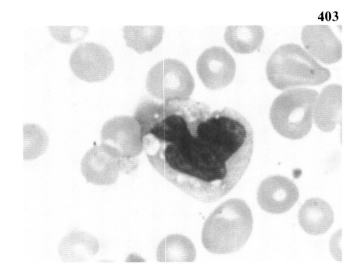

**404** Monocytosis and neutrophilia in a dog with bacterial endocarditis ($\times 40$). The monocytes have vacuolated cytoplasm and abnormal nuclei.

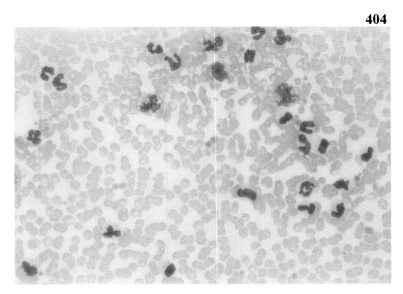

**405** A vacuolated monocyte from a palm civet with chronic infection (monocytes 1.0 $\times 10^9$/l).

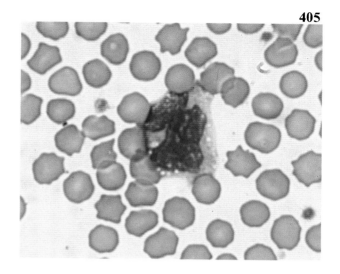

**406** Three abnormal monocytes(?) from a cheetah with *Vaccinia variola* infection. This animal had a marked monocytosis (monocytes 32.6 $\times 10^9$/l). The red cells are crenated. A polychromatic erythroblast showing evidence of retarded nuclear maturation is also present.

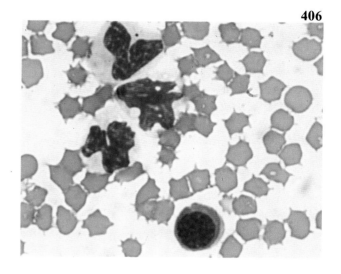

**407** Two atypical monocytes from a gaur with viral enteritis. There is vacuolation of both the cytoplasm and the nuclei (monocytes 2.0 $\times 10^9$/l).

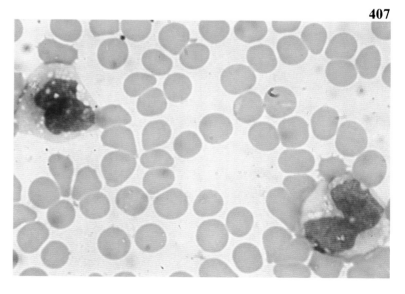

**408** Monocytosis in a cow with acute mastitis (×40).

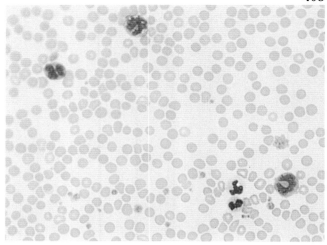

**409** Two atypical monocytes from a guinea pig with lymphadenopathy (monocytes 2.1 × 10$^9$/l).

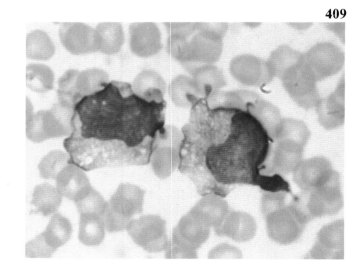

**410** An atypical monocyte with a degenerating nucleus from a Jamaican hutia with chronic eye ulceration and a necrotic lesion of the orbit (monocytes 1.2 × 10$^9$/l).

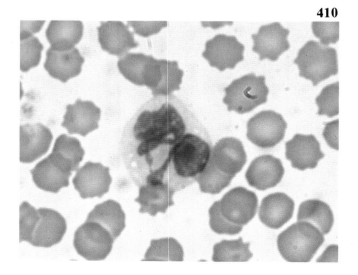

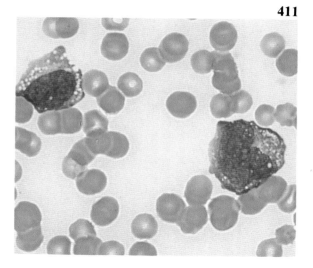

**411** Two pathological monoblasts from a dog with myelomonocytic leukaemia. The red cells show increased rouleaux formation.

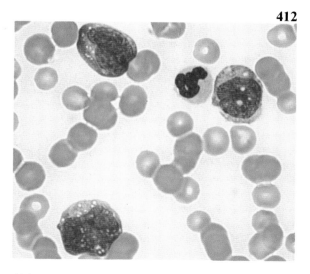

**412** Three pathological monoblasts and a normal neutrophil from the dog in **411**.

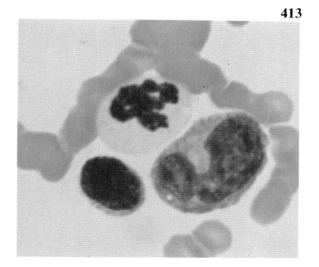

**413** A malignant mononuclear cell in the blood of a horse with neoplasia.

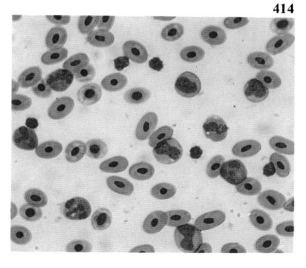

**414** Monocytosis in a black-footed penguin with aspergillosis ($\times 40$, monocytes $3.1 \times 10^9/l$).

**415** Two monocytes, two degranulated heterophils and a lymphocyte with granular cytoplasm from a sarus crane with *Mycobacterium avium* infection (monocytes 5.0 ×10$^9$/l). The monocytes contain small vacuoles and nuclear cleavage is absent. Part of a third monocyte is also present.

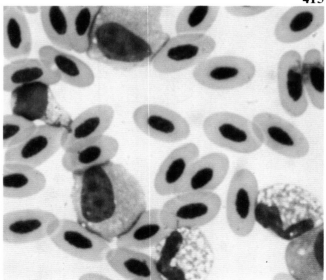

415

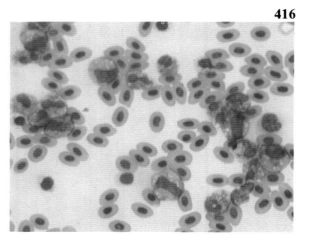

416

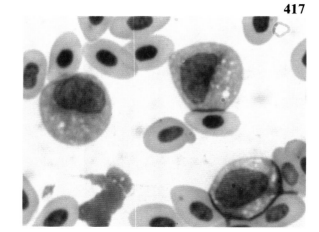

417

**416** Monocytosis and heterophilia in a domestic fowl with *Mycobacterium avium* infection (×40, monocytes 10.1 ×10$^9$/l).

**417** A high power view of three monocytes from the bird in **416**. The cells have cytoplasmic vacuoles and nuclear cleavage is absent.

**418** Monocytosis in an Aldabra giant tortoise suffering from anorexia and muscle wasting (monocytes 1.0 ×10$^9$/l).

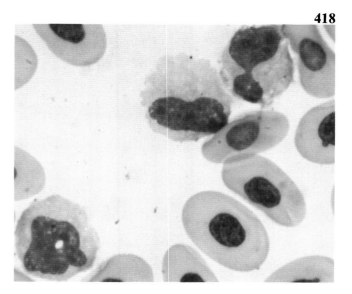

418

**419-422** *Normal azurophil morphology.*

419

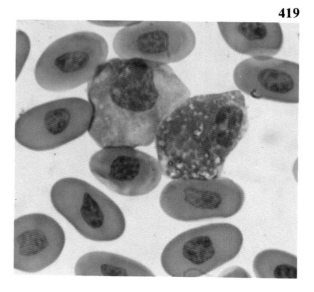

**419** An azurophil and a heterophil from a healthy taipan snake. The azurophil is the cell on the left.

420

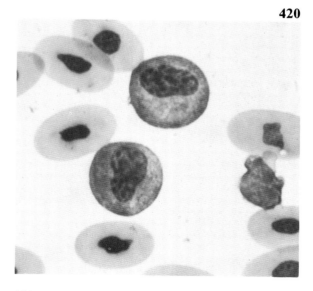

**420** Two azurophils from a healthy reticulated python.

421

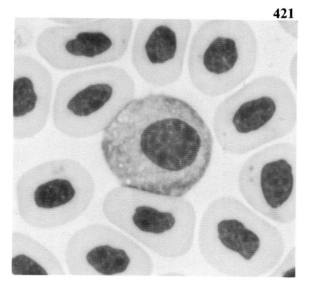

**421** An azurophil with a large amount of cytoplasm from a healthy black-pointed tegu.

422

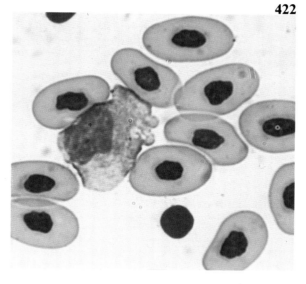

**422** A monocytoid azurophil from a healthy common iguana.

**423-438** *Abnormal azurophils.*

**423** General view of a blood film showing azurophilia and heterophilia in an Eastern fox snake with severe spreading necrosis of the tail (×40, azurophils 20.9 ×10⁹/l). The azurophils have monocytoid nuclei and a tendency for vacuolation.

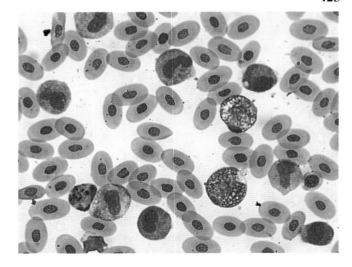

**423**

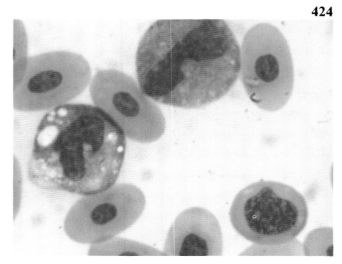

**424**

**424** A higher magnification of two azurophils and a polychromatic erythroblast from the snake in **423**.

**425** Two more large azurophils with excessive cytoplasm from the snake in **423**. In one of the cells, the cytoplasm appears to have shrunk away from the cell membrane. A normal lymphocyte is also present.

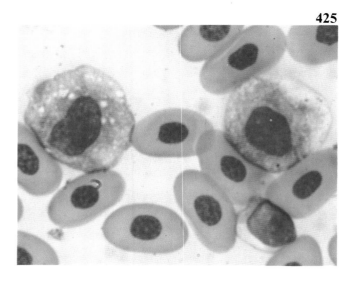

**425**

**426** A highly vacuolated azurophil and a normal thrombocyte from a brown python with stomatitis and respiratory infection (azurophils $4.1 \times 10^9/l$). The cytoplasm of the azurophil contains a few abnormal granules and the cell membrane is scalloped.

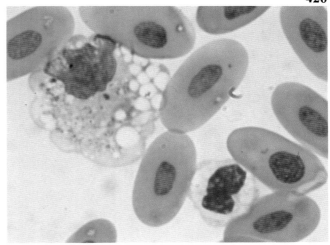

**427** An azurophil, a heterophil and a thrombocyte from the python in **426**. The azurophil has a scalloped cell membrane, cytoplasmic vacuolation and granulation, the latter possibly consisting of phagocytosed material.

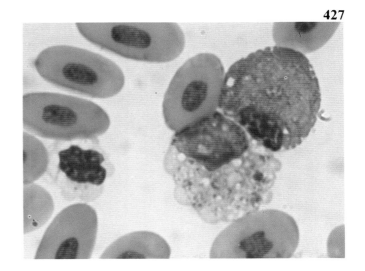

**428** Azurophilia in a carpet python with multiple abscesses, cellulitis and muscle necrosis (azurophils $5.5 \times 10^9/l$). The nuclei show excessive lobulation.

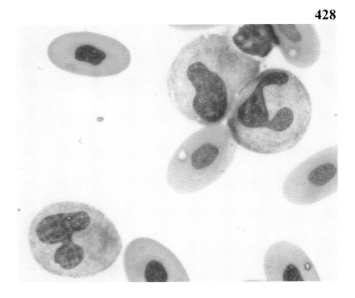

**429** A monocytoid azurophil containing round, blue-staining cytoplasmic inclusion bodies from a Gaboon viper with wasting disease. The lymphocyte and thrombocyte present in the field are normal but the red cell nuclei are deformed.

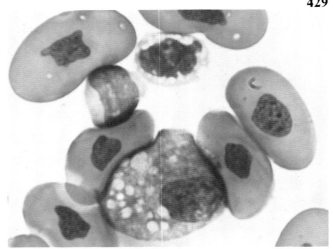

**430** A lymphocytoid azurophil with cytoplasmic inclusions and a normal thrombocyte from the snake in **429**.

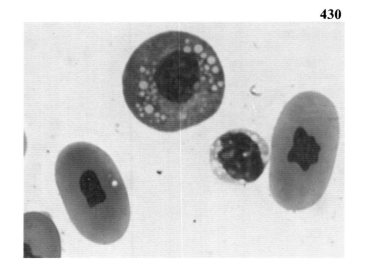

**431** A disrupted azurophil from the snake in **429** showing release of the blue cytoplasmic inclusion bodies.

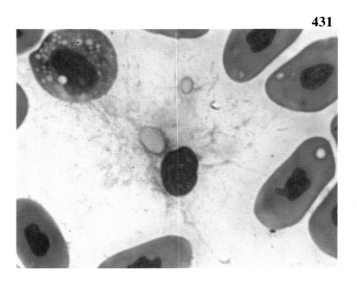

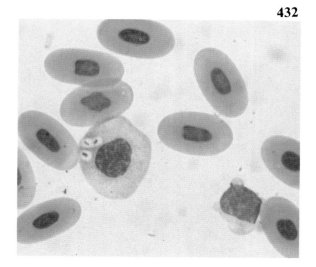

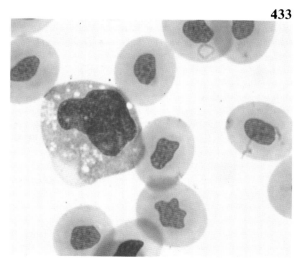

**432** An azurophil with cytoplasmic inclusions (bacteria?) from an Indian python with a facial abscess (azurophils 1.5 $\times 10^9$/l).

**433** A large azurophil with an irregular nucleus and vacuolated cytoplasm from a Montpelier snake suffering from ascites, skin lesions and cloacal haemorrhage. This snake had marked azurophilia (azurophils 13.4 $\times 10^9$/l) and was severely anaemic.

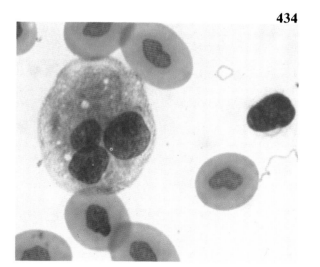

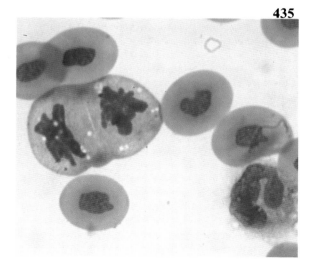

**434, 435** A trinucleated azurophil and an azurophil in mitosis from the snake in **433**. The possibility that this snake was suffering from a malignancy involving the azurophils was not ruled out.

**436** A large azurophil with a trilobed nucleus from a green water dragon with osteomyelitis (azurophils 3.1 $\times 10^9$/l).

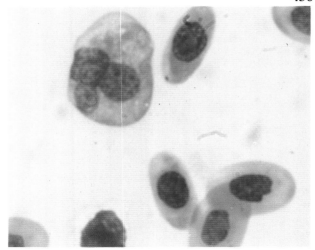

**436**

**437** An azurophil with cytoplasmic budding and a toxic heterophil from a green water dragon with blepharitis (azurophils 7.7 $\times 10^9$/l).

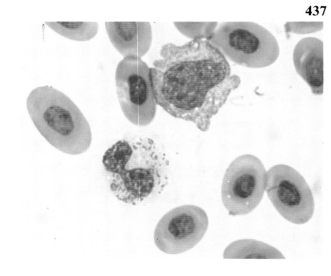

**437**

**438** Two azurophils with intense cytoplasmic granulation from a common iguana with infection associated with a fractured femur (azurophils 0.2 $\times 10^9$/l). The red cells have misshapen nuclei and one cell showing evidence of delayed nuclear maturation is present.

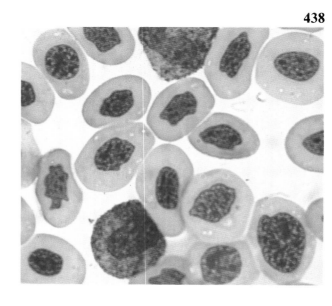

**438**

# *Part 4*
# Normal and Abnormal Platelets and Thrombocytes

By definition, the haemostatic blood cells of all vertebrate animals are correctly described as thrombocytes. In mammals, however, these cells are often referred to as platelets in order to take account of the striking morphological differences which distinguish them from the thrombocytes of other vertebrates. Strictly speaking, platelets are not true cells as they do not contain a nucleus. They are the smallest elements in the circulating blood and are formed from the cytoplasm of megakaryocytes, mainly in the bone marrow, where each megakaryocyte gives rise to several thousand platelets. Interspecies differences in platelet number, size and granularity occur and, as a general rule, there is an inverse relationship between platelet size and platelet count.

In contrast, the thrombocytes of birds and reptiles are significantly larger than mammalian platelets and are nucleated. They are produced from mononuclear precursors in the bone marrow. Non-activated thrombocytes may be oval, spindle-shaped or round with a round or oval, comparatively dense nucleus and clear, blue-grey cytoplasm in which one or two small basophilic granules may be visible. In some avian and particularly in some reptilian species, it can be difficult to distinguish between thrombocytes and lymphocytes and, without experience, there is sometimes confusion between disrupted red cell nuclei and thrombocytes.

Although the stimuli for adhesion and aggregation may be different, platelets and thrombocytes appear to function similarly in haemostasis. The propensity for these cells to become activated by contact with foreign surfaces is an integral part of their haemostatic function but also gives rise to artefactual changes in their morphology in all but the most carefully collected blood samples. The morphological changes associated with platelet activation include spreading, pseudopodial formation, vacuolation, aggregation and loss of granules. Thrombocyte activation leads to cytoplasmic vacuolation, alterations in outline and aggregation. Although, in practice, a small degree of activation often facilitates the correct identification of thrombocytes, it can also obscure clinically significant quantitative and morphological changes.

On films prepared from correctly collected blood samples, thrombocytopenia can be diagnosed from a lack of platelets and the presence of activated platelets or thrombocytes is an indication of disseminated intravascular coagulation. Thrombocytosis occurs as a response to haemorrhage or bacterial infection. Platelet anisocytosis and the presence of giant forms is often associated with myeloid and lymphoid hyperplasia.

**439-455** *Normal variation in platelet and thrombocyte morphology.*

439

**439** Normal platelets from a dog. Pseudopodium formation and the tendency for platelets to aggregate together is shown. These changes represent the first stage of platelet activation during sample collection.

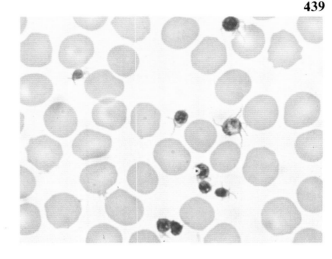

**440**

**440** Platelet anisocytosis in a normal moose. Pseudopodium formation is evident.

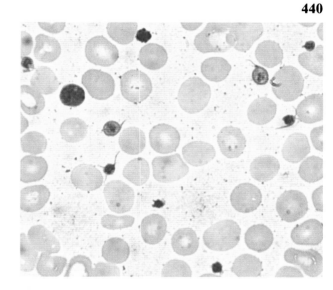

**441**

**441** Aggregated platelets in a badly collected blood sample from a goat (×40).

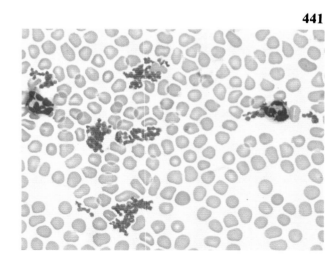

**442** Two different morphological types of platelets from a guinea pig. The filamentous platelets are unusual but apparently normal in a few species of mammals. They may represent a more easily activated sub-population.

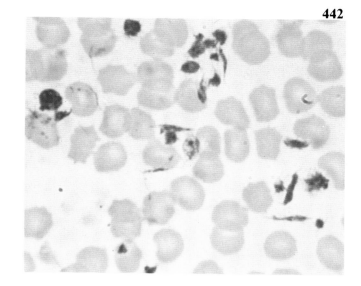
442

**443** Normal and filamentous platelets from a healthy Bruijn's echidna.

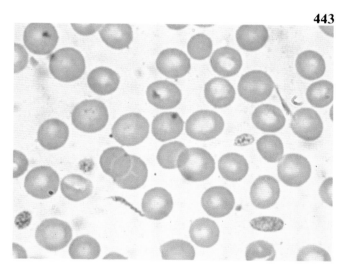
443

**444** Photomicrographs at the same magnification of platelet-rich human plasma (left) and thrombocyte-rich domestic fowl plasma showing the difference in cell size. Thrombocytes are larger than platelets but occur in smaller numbers so that the packed thrombocyte volume and the packed platelet volume are similar. One red cell is present in the domestic fowl sample.

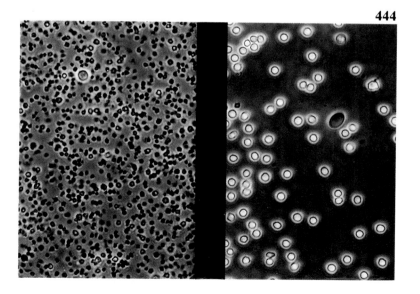
444

**445** SEM of aggregated platelets from an anubis baboon (left) and aggregated thrombocytes from a domestic turkey showing structural similarities.

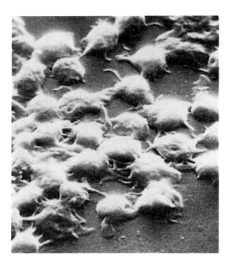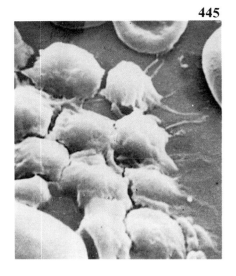

**446** Two spindle-shaped thrombocytes from a normal kori bustard.

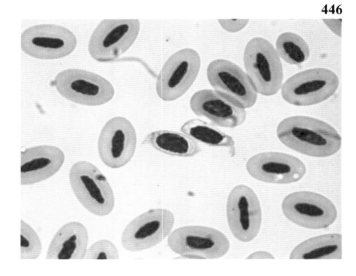

**447** Spindle-shaped thrombocytes from a rosy flamingo.

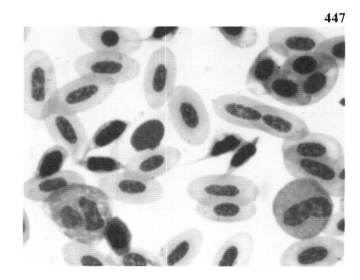

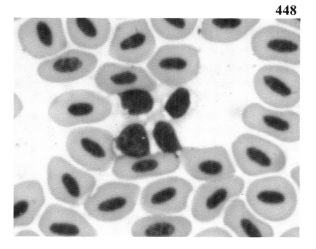

**448**

**448** An aggregate of four normal thrombocytes from a moorhen.

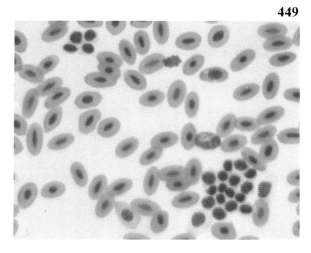

**449**

**449** Thrombocyte aggregates from an ostrich (×40).

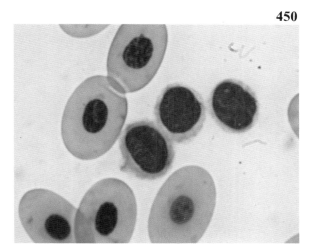

**450**

**450** Three normal thrombocytes from a Hermann's tortoise. These cells could be misidentified as lymphocytes but are smaller and have denser nuclei. The thrombocytes seen here show some evidence of aggregation.

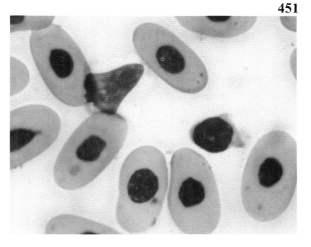

**451**

**451** A thrombocyte and a lymphocyte from a spur-thighed tortoise. In this animal the distinction between the two cell types is obvious.

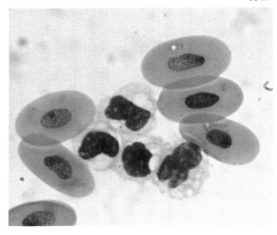

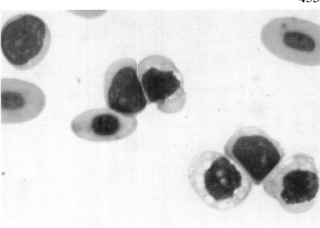

**452** An aggregate of four thrombocytes with vacuolated cytoplasm and irregular nuclei from a brown python.

**453** Three thrombocytes and three lymphocytes from an Indian python. The thrombocytes have smaller nuclei and less regular cytoplasm.

454

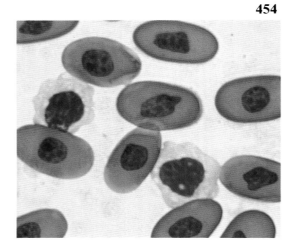

**454** Two normal thrombocytes from a taipan snake. The cytoplasm of the cells has an irregular foamy appearance associated with partial activation.

455

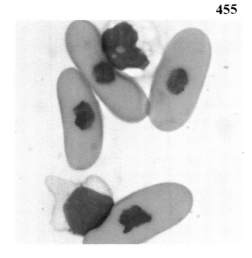

**455** A thrombocyte and a lymphocyte from a Chinese alligator. The thrombocyte is at the top of the field.

**456-465** *Variations in platelets and thrombocytes associated with disease.*

**456** A greatly increased platelet count (thrombocytosis) in a casiragua with infected fight wounds (platelets 1370 $\times 10^9/l$). A raised platelet count is found in association with bacterial infection in many mammalian species. This animal also had neutrophilia and monocytosis.

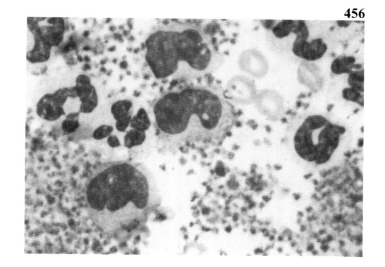

**457** Thrombocytosis and neutrophilia in a plains viscacha with acute inflammatory disease (platelets 902 $\times 10^9/l$). One giant platelet is present.

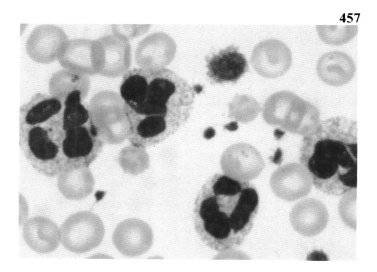

**458** Thrombocytosis with 'shift' platelets in a dog, following rupture of a splenic haemangiosarcoma with intraperitoneal haemorrhage. The red cells show poikilocytosis and schistocytosis.

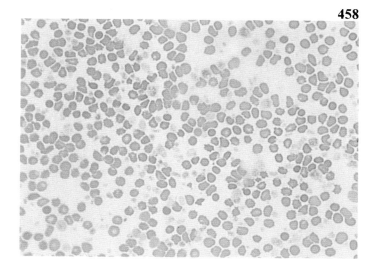

**459** Two partially activated giant platelets from a dog with thrombocytopenia associated with lymphoma (platelets $15 \times 10^9$/l).

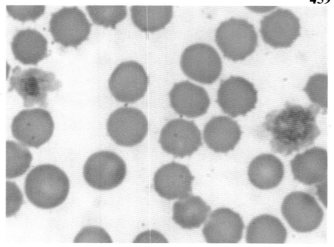

**459**

**460** Giant platelets from a dog with lymphoma, on steroid treatment.

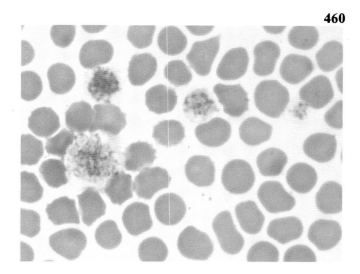

**460**

**461** Giant platelets from a dog with anaemia and a hormonal imbalance (platelets $233 \times 10^9$/l). The red cells show anisocytosis and a neutrophil showing a right shift and cytoplasmic vacuoles is present.

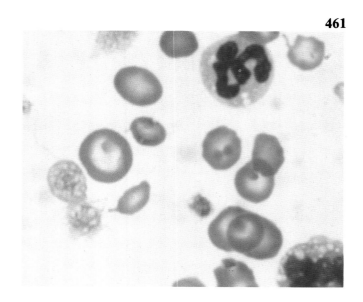

**461**

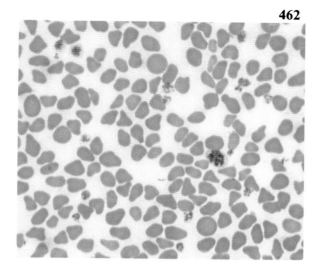

**462** A giant platelet with distinctive granulation from a markhor with vitamin E deficiency. Triangular red cells occur normally as an *in vitro* artefact in this species.

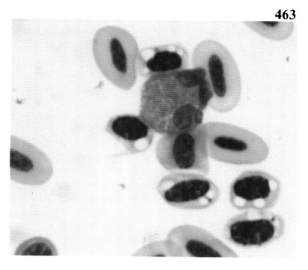

**463** Vacuolated thrombocytes from a golden eagle with regenerative anaemia. This bird had a relatively high thrombocyte count (61 $\times 10^9$/l). The intact appearance of the thrombocyte membranes suggests that vacuolation may not be caused by activation in this case.

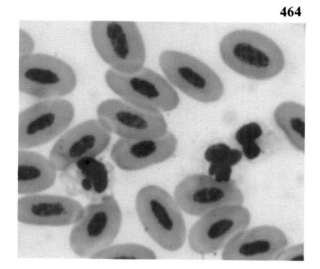

**464** Thrombocytes with polymorphic nuclei from an African grey parrot with a respiratory infection (thrombocytes 9 $\times 10^9$/l).

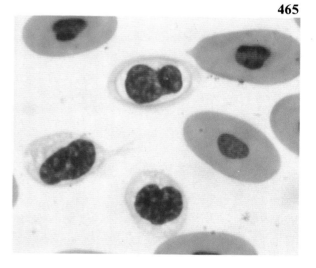

**465** Thrombocytes with slightly polymorphic nuclei from a reticulated python suffering from anorexia and severe, chronic stomatitis.

# *Part 5* **Blood Parasites**

## *M.A. Peirce*

To the inexperienced observer, there are many artefacts occurring in blood and tissue smears which can be mistaken for parasites and the converse is also true. For diagnostic and taxonomic purposes, it is essential to avoid contamination of the smears with dust and other particles and with stain precipitate. Whenever possible, the smears should be freshly prepared from living animals as artefacts caused by disintegrating cells and contaminants are found more frequently in anticoagulated and *post mortem* blood samples; distortion of any parasites present may take place under these circumstances.

In this section, a wide spectrum of blood parasite species in their normal morphological forms is presented. The majority of slides were prepared from living animals with natural infections. The material was obtained either from clinical cases or from surveys. In a few instances, experimental material has been included for the sake of morphological clarity. A few examples are shown of parasites in *post mortem* and anticoagulated blood samples in order to demonstrate some of the problems which can occur.

**466**

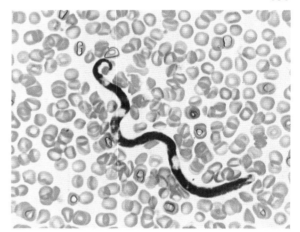

**466** Microfilarian in blood from a newly captured capuchin monkey (×40).

**467**

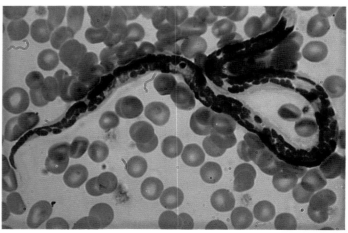

**467** Microfilarian from a newly captured squirrel monkey.

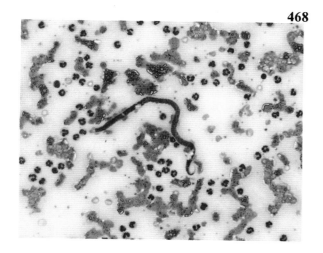

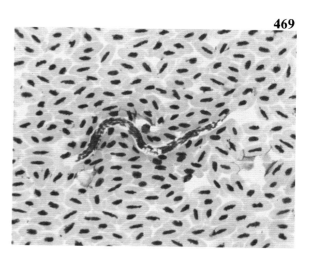

**468** *Dirofilaria immitis* (heart worm) microfilarian from a dog (buffy coat preparation). This organism has a cosmopolitan distribution in dogs, cats and foxes and is frequently pathogenic due to the presence of a large number of adult worms.

**469** *Chandlerella sinensis* microfilarian from a red-billed blue magpie (×40).

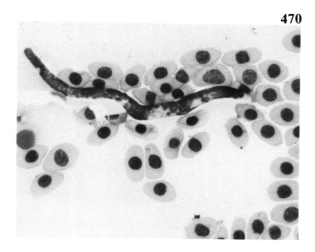

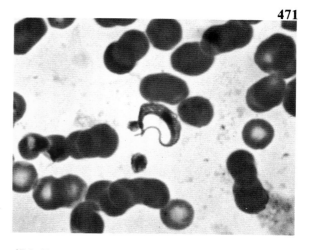

**470** A microfilarian from a greater plated lizard (×40).

**471** *Trypanosoma cruzi*, the cause of Chagas' disease in the New World where it has been recorded in numerous species of mammals. It may be pathogenic in dogs and cats but there is little evidence of this in wildlife.

**472** *Trypanosoma evansi*, the cause of 'Surra' in camels, equids, Asian elephants, dogs and other domestic and wild mammals throughout a wide distribution in hot and warm-temperate climates. Pathogenicity depends upon the virulence of the parasite strain.

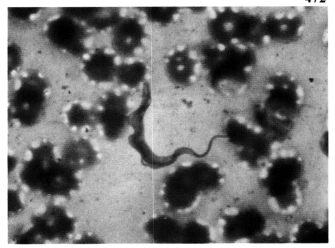

**473** *Trypanosoma equiperdum*, the cause of 'Dourine', a venereal disease of equids. This organism is widespread and is more pathogenic in horses than in donkeys or mules. The parasites are found only rarely in the bloodstream.

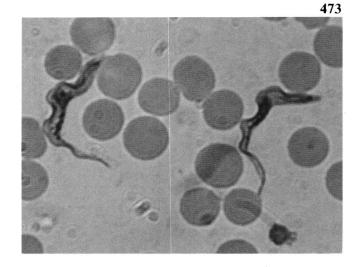

**474** *Trypanosoma brucei*, a polymorphic salivarian trypanosome of Africa where it is highly pathogenic and frequently fatal in domestic mammals, particularly horses. The parasite is found in a large number of wild mammal reservoir hosts, especially antelopes.

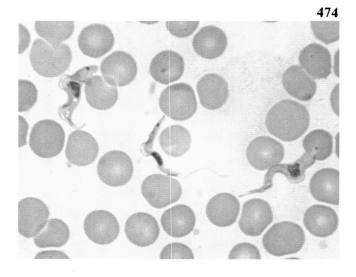

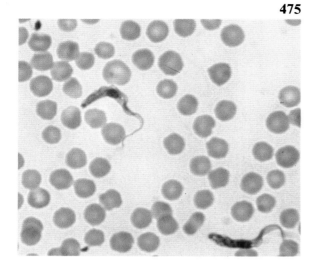

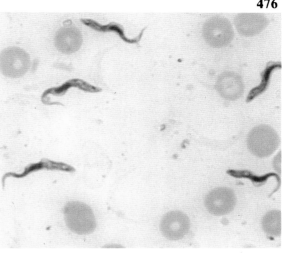

**475** *Trypanosoma vivax*, the cause of 'Souma' in Africa and, to a lesser extent, in central-south America, the West Indies and Mauritius where it is pathogenic in domestic mammals, particularly in ungulates. The reservoir hosts are wild mammals, especially antelopes.

**476** *Trypanosoma congolense*, an African species highly pathogenic in domestic mammals and common in wild ruminants. Pathogenicity depends upon the virulence of the parasite strain.

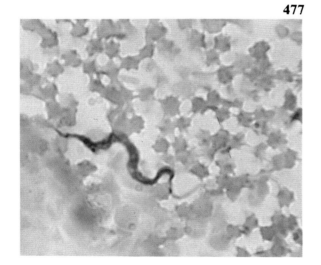

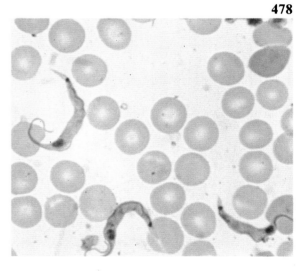

**477** *Trypanosoma theileri*, a parasite with a world-wide distribution in cattle, also occurs in European bison and in African antelopes; generally considered to be non-pathogenic.

**478** *Trypanosoma lewisi*, a parasite with a world-wide distribution in rats; generally considered to be non-pathogenic.

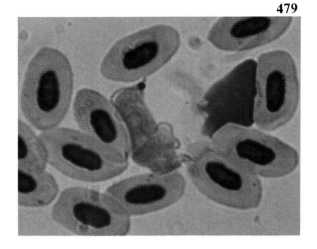

**479** *Trypanosoma everetti* from a blue tit. This is a small trypanosome, occurring in a wide range of avian hosts in Europe, Africa and probably Asia. It is not known to be pathogenic.

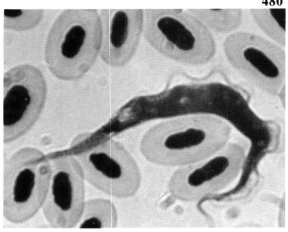

**480** *Trypanosoma pycnonoti* from a white-eared bulbul. This is a non-pathogenic species occurring in African bulbuls.

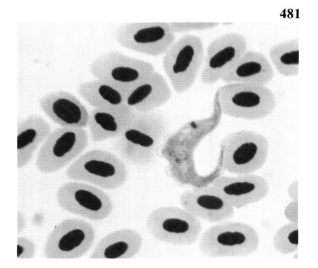

**481** *Trypanosoma bouffardi* from a blue waxbill. This is a non-pathogenic species occurring in African passerines.

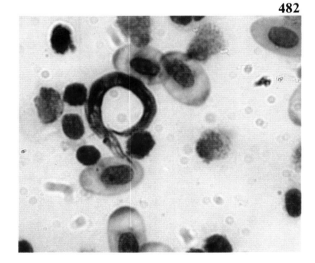

**482** *Trypanosoma avium* from a fish owl (buffy coat preparation). This species has a world-wide distribution in Strigiformes and possibly occurs in other avian groups.

**483** *Leishmania donovani* in white cells from a dog in which it is pathogenic although rarely fatal (bone marrow smear).

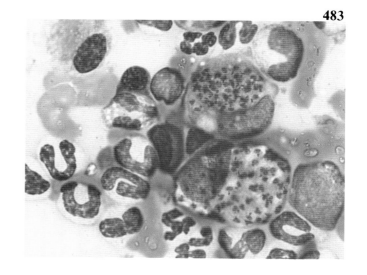

**484** *Leucocytozoon ziemanni* macrogametocyte in an erythrocyte from a little owl. This parasite occurs world-wide in Strigiformes but is not known to be pathogenic.

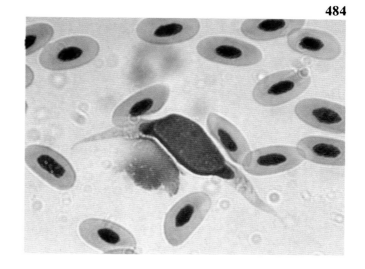

**485** A distorted microgametocyte of *L. ziemanni* in an EDTA blood sample from a tawny owl.

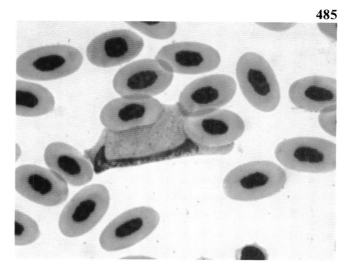

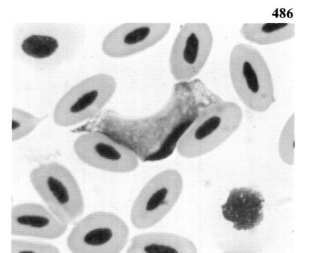

**486** *Leucocytozoon* sp. macrogametocyte from a mikado pheasant.

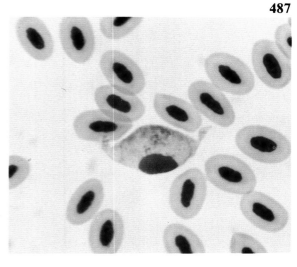

**487** *Leucocytozoon balmorali* microgametocyte (elongate form) in a puffback shrike erythrocyte. This organism is not known to be pathogenic.

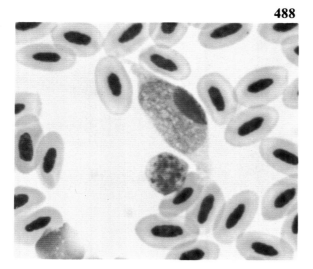

**488** *L. balmorali* macrogametocyte (elongate form) from a puffback shrike.

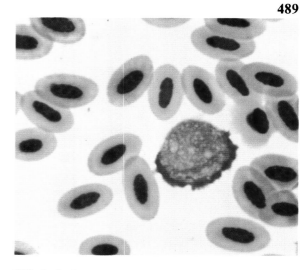

**489** *L. balmorali* macrogametocyte (round form) from a puffback shrike.

**490** *Leucocytozoon toddi* macrogameto-cyte from a goshawk. This organism is not known to be pathogenic although high para-sitaemias frequently occur in chicks of some Accipitridae. It has a world-wide distribution.

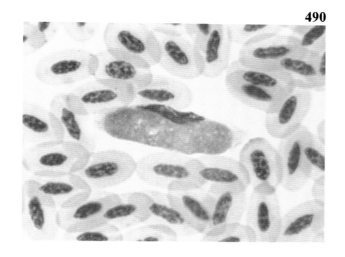

**490**

**491** Three distorted *L. toddi* macrogameto-cytes from a goshawk (×40).

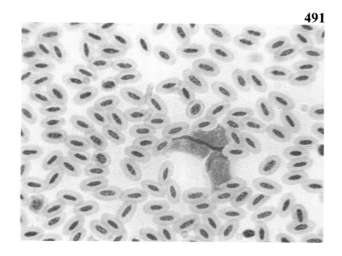

**491**

**492** *Leucocytozoon naevei* macrogameto-cyte from a yellow-necked spurfowl. This parasite is common in African Phasianidae but there is no evidence of pathogenicity.

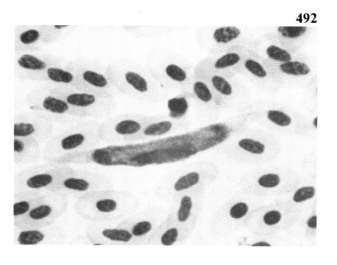

**492**

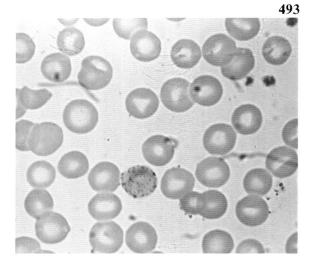

**493** *Plasmodium brasilianum* macrogametocyte from a newly imported squirrel monkey. This is a pathogenic parasite occurring in New World monkeys.

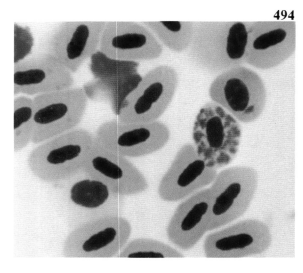

**494** *Plasmodium circumflexum* schizont from a blue waxbill. This organism has a cosmopolitan distribution in passerines and is also found in grouse, geese and waders. It is mildly pathogenic in its natural hosts.

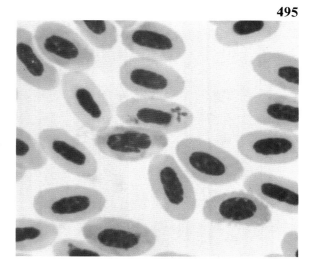

**495** *Plasmodium rouxi* schizont from a dark plain-backed pipit. The parasite is common in Africa and Asia and has been recorded less often in Europe and USA. It occurs more frequently in passerines than in other avian orders and may be mildly pathogenic in its natural hosts.

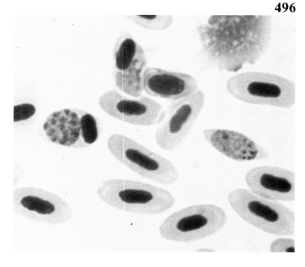

**496** *Plasmodium relictum*, a parasite with world-wide distribution in many avian families, in some of which it is pathogenic and often fatal.

**497** *Plasmodium gallinaceum* from a domestic fowl. The natural host in Asia is the jungle fowl in which it is non-pathogenic. In domestic fowl it may be highly pathogenic.

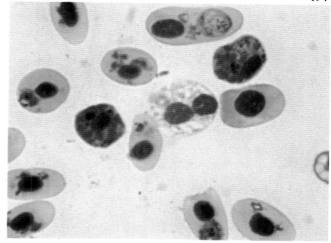

**497**

**498** *Plasmodium* sp. trophozoites from a wattled starling (*post mortem* sample). There are two erythroplastids in the field.

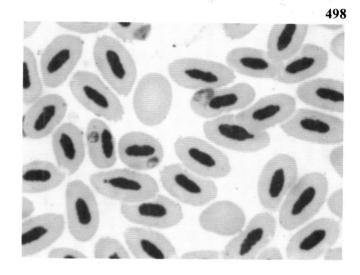

**498**

**499** *Plasmodium* sp. trophozoites in an EDTA blood sample from a snowy owl.

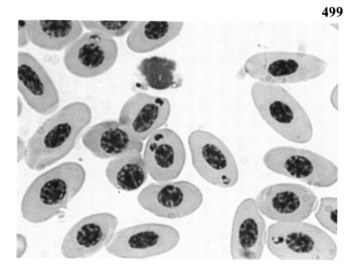

**499**

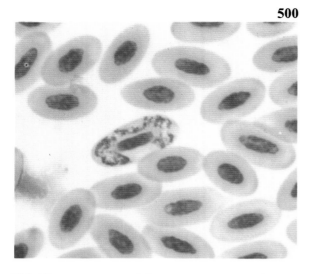

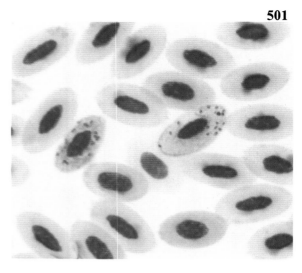

**500** *Haemoproteus nisi* macrogametocyte from a sparrowhawk. Note the reddish-purple volutin granules in the parasite cytoplasm. This species is not known to be pathogenic.

**501** Macrogametocyte and microgametocyte of *H. nisi* from a sparrowhawk.

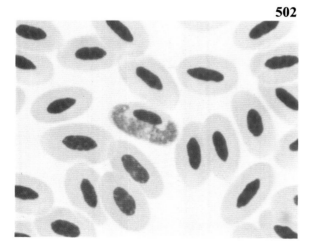

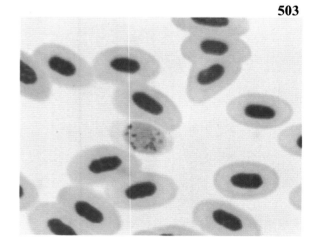

**502** *Haemoproteus columbae* macrogametocyte from a Cape turtle dove. This parasite has a cosmopolitan distribution in Columbiformes and is reported to be pathogenic in young pigeons.

**503** *Haemoproteus sequeirae* macrogametocyte in an enucleated erythrocyte of a scarlet-chested sunbird. This is a non-pathogenic species occurring in Nectariniidae.

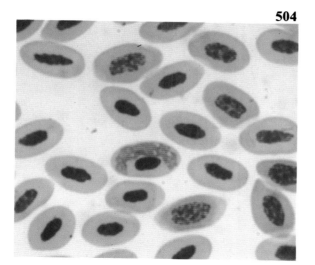

**504** *Haemoproteus handai* macrogametocyte from a Moluccan cockatoo. The parasite occurs in Asian and Australasian psittacines and is not known to be pathogenic although high parasitaemias may cause anaemia.

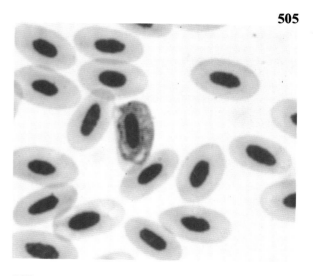

**505** *Haemoproteus* sp. macrogametocyte from a blue and gold macaw.

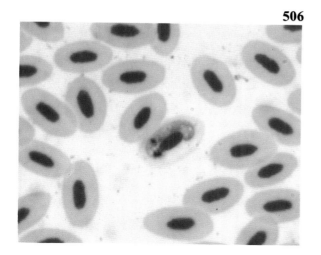

**506** *Haemoproteus* sp. macrogametocyte from an African grey parrot.

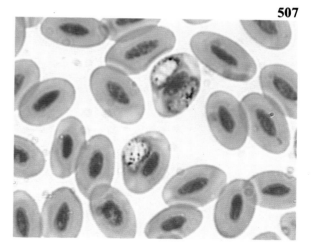

**507** Distorted *Haemoproteus crumenium* parasites in an EDTA blood sample from a healthy marabou stork.

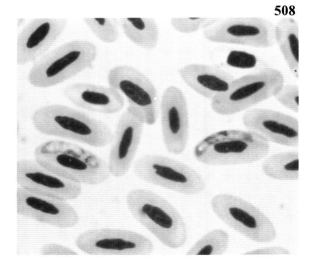

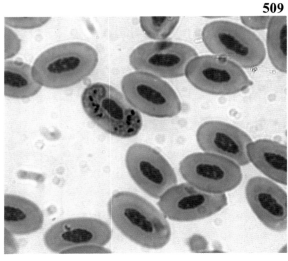

**508** Macrogametocyte and microgametocyte of *Haemoproteus balearicae* from a crowned crane. This organism is not known to be pathogenic.

**509** *Haemoproteus* sp. from a snowy owl.

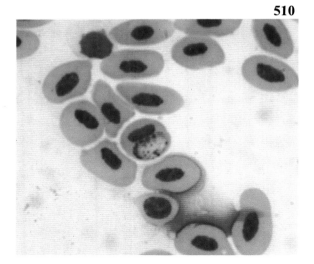

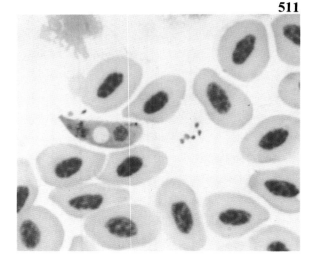

**510** Distorted *Haemoproteus* sp. in an EDTA blood sample from a tawny owl.

**511** *Haemoproteus* sp. ookinete in a 48-hour-old EDTA blood sample from a tawny owl. This stage normally occurs in the vector but may be seen occasionally in blood samples maintained at ambient temperatures for sufficient time to permit development.

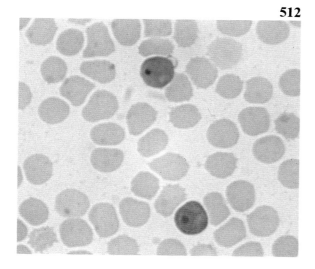

**512** *Hepatocystis epomophori* macrogametocyte and microgametocyte from a fruit bat. This parasite is not known to be pathogenic.

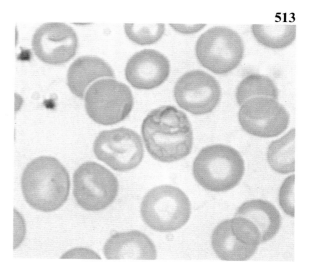

**513** *Hepatocystis kochi* immature gametocyte from a vervet monkey. This parasite occurs in guenons and other African monkeys and is mildly pathogenic but non-fatal.

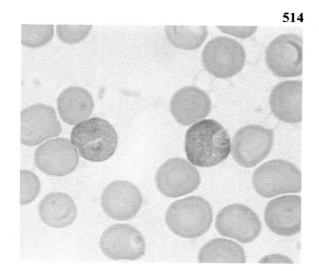

**514** Mature gametocytes of *H.kochi* from a vervet monkey.

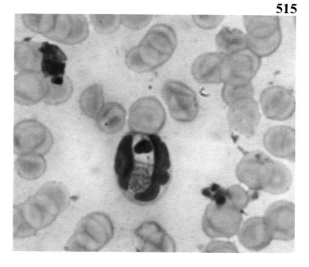

**515** *Hepatozoon sciuri* in a white blood cell from a grey squirrel. The parasite is non-pathogenic.

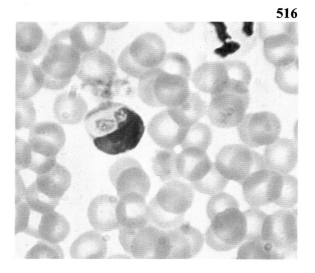

**516** *Hepatozoon canis* in a white blood cell from a dog. The parasite has a world-wide distribution in dogs and wild canids. In dogs it is usually pathogenic and often fatal.

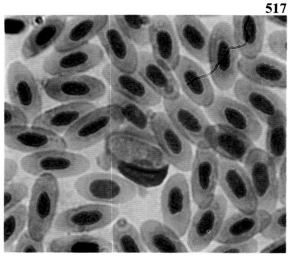

**517** *Hepatozoon albatrossi* in a mononuclear white cell from a wandering albatross. The parasite is not known to be pathogenic.

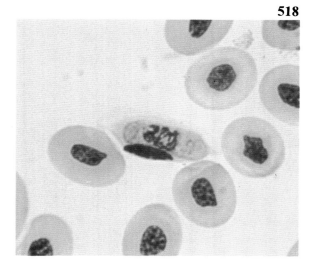

**518** *Hepatozoon boodoni* in a Zambian house snake red cell. The parasite is not known to be pathogenic.

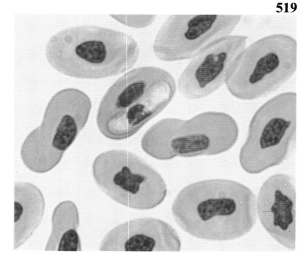

**519** *Haemogregarina sebai* from an African python. The parasite is not known to be pathogenic.

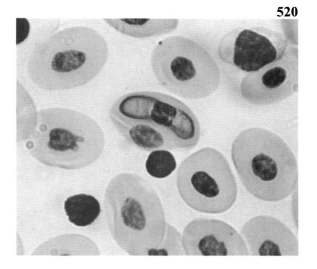

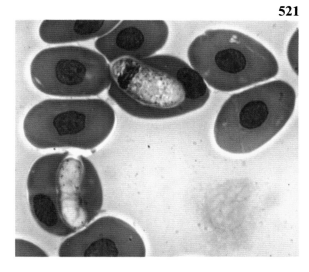

**520** *Haemogregarina musotae* from a Seychelles house snake. This parasite also occurs in other species of house snake on mainland Africa. It is not known to be pathogenic.

**521** *Haemogregarina* sp., probably *H.serpentium*, in a *post mortem* blood sample from an anaconda.

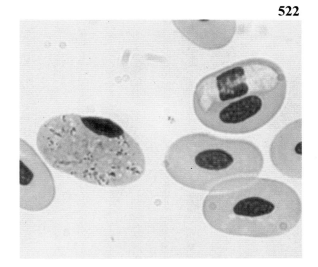

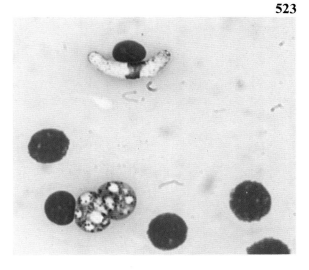

**522** *Haemogregarina najae* and *Haemoproteus mesnili* from a Mozambique spitting cobra. This haemogregarine is widely distributed in African cobras but is not known to be pathogenic.

**523** Distorted haemogregarine and *Haemoproteus* parasites in a haemolysed EDTA blood sample from a yellow-footed tortoise.

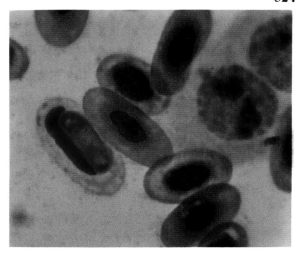

**524** *Karyolysis* sp. in a *post mortem* sample from a green lizard.

**525** *Lankesterella* sp. in a basophilic erythroblast from a house sparrow. The parasite may be pathogenic in young birds.

**526** *Babesia gibsoni* from a dog. The parasite is common in dogs in the Indian sub-continent, China and north Africa and is pathogenic, often fatal. It also occurs in wild canids in which it is non-pathogenic.

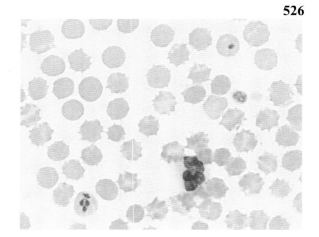

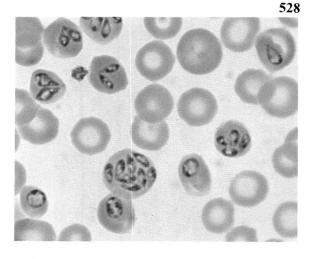

**527** *Babesia canis* chronic infection in a dog. This organism has a cosmopolitan distribution in the dog and wild carnivores and is pathogenic, often fatal.

**528** *B. canis* acute infection in a dog showing multiple divisions in the erythrocytes, leading to severe anaemia.

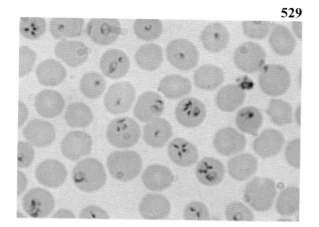

529

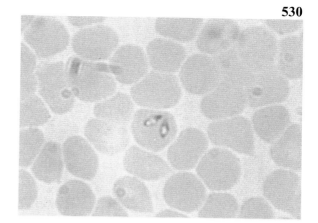

530

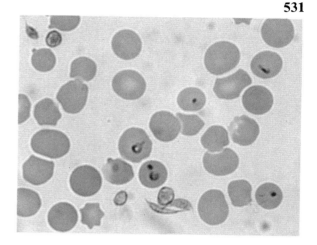

531

**529** *Babesia equi* from a horse. This organism is widely distributed in equids including zebras. In most equids it is pathogenic and frequently fatal although it is not known to be fatal in zebras.

**530** *Babesia caballi* from a horse. Dividing pyriform merozoites are present. The organism is widely distributed in horses, donkeys and mules and is less pathogenic than *B. equi* although it can be fatal.

**531** Acute infection with *B. caballi* from a horse, showing some parasites becoming pyknotic.

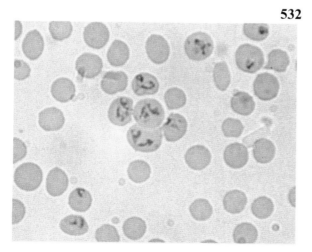

532

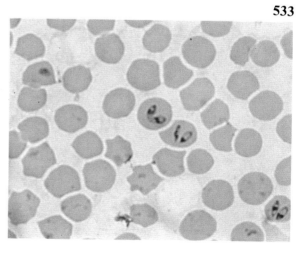

533

**532** *Babesia major* from cattle. This organism is widely distributed in cattle in south America, southern Europe, Great Britain, USSR and parts of north and west Africa. It is also found in bison. Pathogenicity is usually mild, except in bison in which it can be fatal.

**533** *Babesia bigemina* from cattle. This parasite is widely distributed in tropical and sub-tropical regions and is pathogenic with a high mortality in acute cases.

**534**

**535**

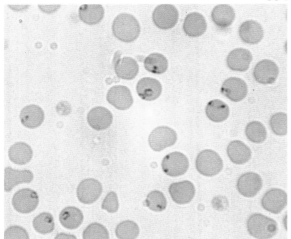

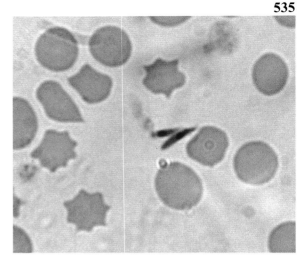

**534** *Babesia divergens* from cattle. The distribution of this parasite is mainly confined to northern Europe where it occurs in cattle and probably also in deer. It is pathogenic and sometimes fatal, with haemoglobinuria giving rise to classical 'Red Water Fever'.

**535** *B. divergens* vermicules in cattle blood from a natural tick-transmitted infection. It is very rare to observe these stages in the blood.

**536**

**537**

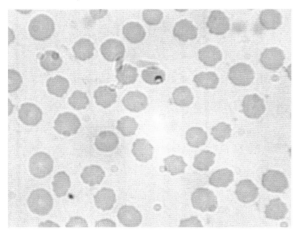

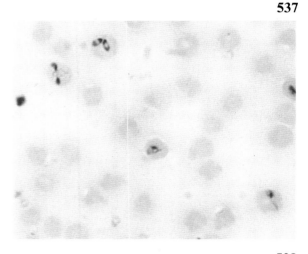

**536** *Babesia ovis* from a sheep. This parasite is widely distributed in sheep and goats and is pathogenic but rarely fatal.

**538**

**537** *Babesia motasi* from a sheep. Also widely distributed in sheep and goats but, compared with *B. ovis*, is larger, more pathogenic and frequently fatal in the acute form.

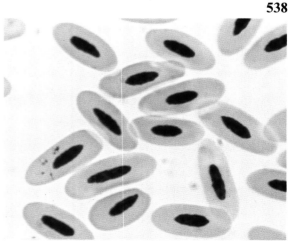

**538** *Babesia balearicae* from a crowned crane. Parasites of the genus *Babesia* are rare in birds although several species have been described. Nothing is known concerning their pathogenicity.

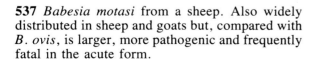

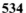

166

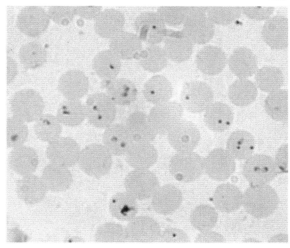

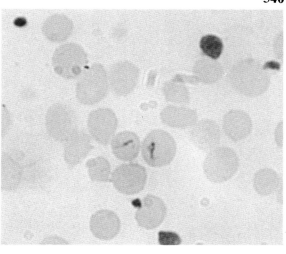

**539** *Theileria parva* (East Coast Fever) from cattle. This intracellular organism is pathogenic with a high mortality in east African cattle but is non-pathogenic in buffalo.

**540** *Theileria orientalis*, the cause of benign bovine theileriosis, has a wide distribution but most strains are only slightly pathogenic and non-fatal. *T. orientalis* is morphologically indistinguishable from *T. mutans* which is now considered to be a strictly African species.

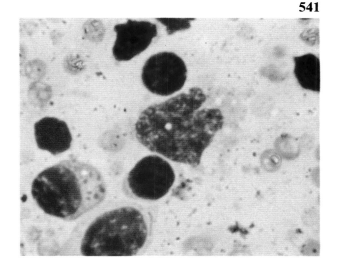

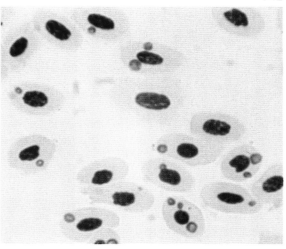

**541** Schizont of *Theileria lestoquardi (T. hirci)* in a lymphocyte from a sheep (lymph node smear). The parasite is widely distributed in sheep and goats and is highly pathogenic, usually fatal, in adult animals.

**542** *Aegyptianella pullorum* from a domestic fowl. This organism occurs in the red cells of domestic ducks, geese and turkeys and may be highly pathogenic, particularly in newly introduced stock. Its distribution follows that of the fowl tick, *Argas persicus*, by which it is transmitted.

**543** *Anaplasma marginale* from an eland. This intracellular parasite has a wide distribution in cattle and wild ungulates. In cattle, pathogenicity increases with age and, in animals older than three years, the disease is often fatal.

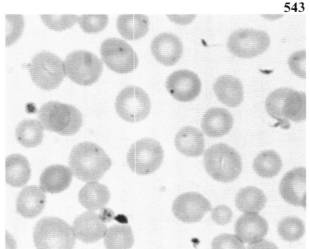
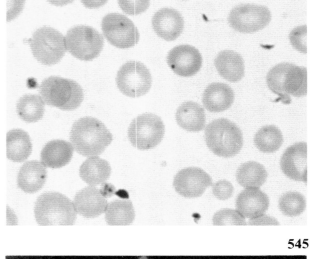

**544**

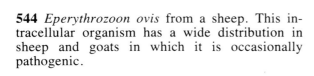
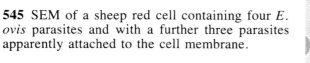

**545**

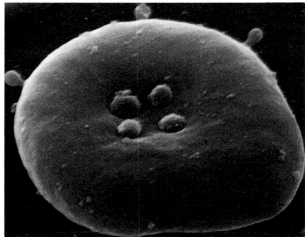

**544** *Eperythrozoon ovis* from a sheep. This intracellular organism has a wide distribution in sheep and goats in which it is occasionally pathogenic.

**545** SEM of a sheep red cell containing four *E. ovis* parasites and with a further three parasites apparently attached to the cell membrane.

**546**

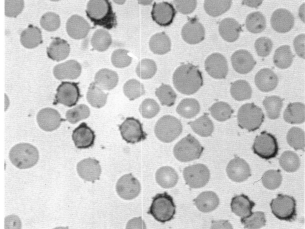

**546** Bovine Eperythrozoonosis. This has a world-wide distribution in cattle and may be mildly pathogenic although rarely fatal.

**547** *Ehrlichia (=Cytoecetes) phagocytophilia* from cattle, the cause of bovine and ovine tick-borne fever in Europe. The parasite occurs as a morula in leucocytes. The disease is generally of low pathogenicity and is rarely fatal although it may cause abortion and a drop in milk yield.

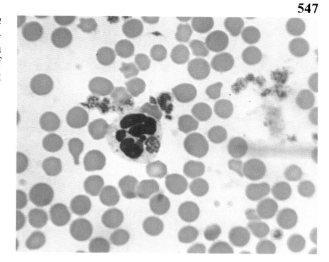

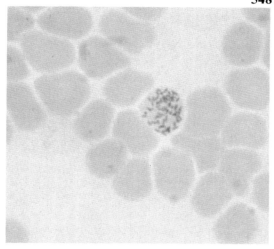

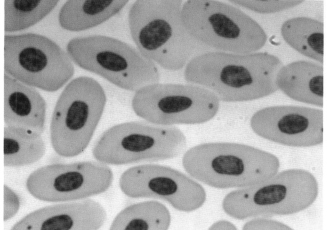

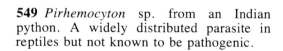

**548** *Grahamella* sp. from a giant rat. This organism occurs commonly in many species of small mammals world-wide. It is not known to be pathogenic.

**549** *Pirhemocyton* sp. from an Indian python. A widely distributed parasite in reptiles but not known to be pathogenic.

**550** Rickettsia-like organisms, morphologically resembling *Pirhemocyton*, in the blood of an olive thrush. Similar organisms are frequently encountered in avian hosts.

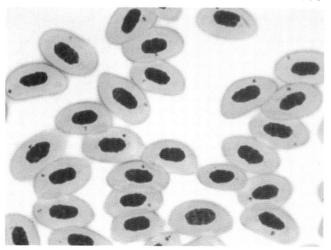

# *Appendix*
# Haematological and Photographic Techniques

## HAEMATOLOGICAL TECHNIQUES

Blood films for examination of cell morphology were prepared from samples of venous blood collected into commercially available plastic tubes containing the potassium salt of ethylene diamine tetra-acetic acid (2K EDTA, sequestrene) at a concentration of 1.5mg per ml of blood. After air-drying, the films were fixed in absolute methanol for two minutes and stained by the May-Grünwald-Giemsa technique. Blood films illustrating the presence of parasites were prepared mainly from fresh, non-anticoagulated blood samples and were stained with Giemsa stain. Reticulocytes and Heinz bodies were stained supravitally with new methylene blue. Microscopic examinations were carried out using a ×40 and ×100 (oil immersion) objective.

## PHOTOGRAPHIC TECHNIQUES

The majority of the illustrations in this Atlas were made with the 35 mm camera attachment of a Zeiss Ultraphot II Photomicroscope, equipped with a 100 wt 12 volt tungsten filament lamp (colour/temperature 3150 K) and an electronic microflash unit (Zeiss U.N. 60, colour/temperature 5500K). The microscope was fitted with a Zeiss Planapochromat, flat field oil immersion objective ×100 (projective 3.2/Optivar 1.25). A colourless immersion oil of RI 1.515 was used and all blood films were mounted for photography.

Colour reversal (slide) film was employed throughout, comprising mainly Kodak Kodachrome II Professional (ASA 25 and 64), Ektachrome 50 (tungsten), Fuji 50 and Agfachrome 50. All films were bulk purchased and of the same emulsion number to minimise batch to batch variation.

Basic colour temperature corrections were needed for all films. Cokin 80 and 82 series polycarbonate camera filters and Lee CTB or CTO acetate gels were mainly used for this purpose. Cokin polycarbonate filters are lightweight, unbreakable and of high optical quality and can be used in place of the more expensive glass filters for all applications except those involving very high temperature lamps. Lee light-control filters are available in rolls and sheets designed for use in the theatrical and television lighting industry. They are widely used in many areas of photography and provide the photomicrographer with a robust and inexpensive replacement for gelatine filters.

A colour compensation filter CCIOY was required to correct the blue bias of the electronic flash. Additionally, an Ealing Beck didymium filter (part no. 26/3061, 50.8 × 50.8mm × 2mm) was used to improve the colour reproduction on Kodachrome films.

Film calibration tests were carried out to determine the basic emulsion characteristics under the pertaining working conditions. Test films were mounted and bound together to provide a permanent set of reference standards (a 'Ring-a-Round') which could be used to determine colour casts and any further filter corrections which appeared necessary (**551-562**).

A colour-corrected light box and Kodak print viewing filters were used for examining the colour transparencies and basic colour correction was then carried out using the appropriate Ilford Cibachrome colour printing filters which were fitted under the substage condenser of the microscope.

**551-562** *A typical exposure colour correction 'Ring-a-Round'.*

A systematic series such as this provides an economical means of assessing and monitoring the different variables in colour photomicrography. Variation of colour temperature caused by lamp ageing or voltage fluctuations can be corrected quickly by reference to such a chart:

*refers to exposure settings on a Zeiss ultraphot photomicroscope

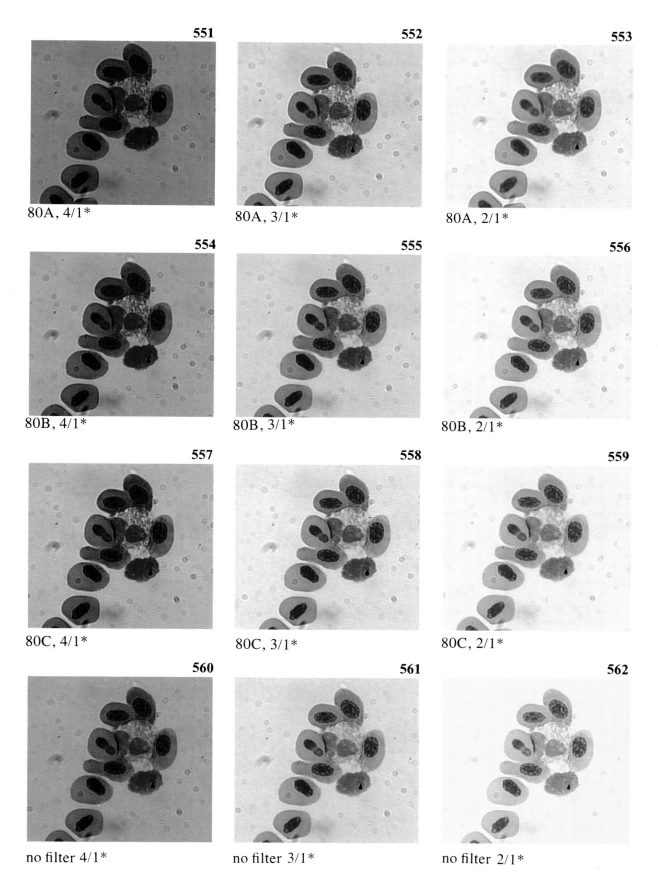

551

80A, 4/1*

552

80A, 3/1*

553

80A, 2/1*

554

80B, 4/1*

555

80B, 3/1*

556

80B, 2/1*

557

80C, 4/1*

558

80C, 3/1*

559

80C, 2/1*

560

no filter 4/1*

561

no filter 3/1*

562

no filter 2/1*

171

For some blood films, subtle differences in staining required modification to both colour and exposure levels in order to obtain optimum reproduction. A bracketed series of exposures through weak colour filters, CCIOR, CCIOG, CCIOY, CCIOB, CCIOM and CCIOC is helpful with this and produces a range of variations in the colours of the cells without any obvious colour cast.

**563-564** *Basic data for correction of colour reproduction.*

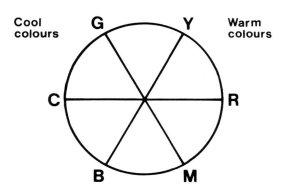

563

| Cast ↓ Add | YELLOW ↓ (M+C) Blue | MAGENTA ↓ (Y+C) Green | CYAN ↓ (Y+M) Red |
|---|---|---|---|
| Cast Add | RED (Y+M) ↓ Cyan | GREEN (Y+C) ↓ Magenta | BLUE (M+C) ↓ Yellow |

**563** Any one colour is made up of the two colours adjacent to it, e.g. Red M Y Green C Y Blue C M. Complementary colours cancel each other out, thus colour casts can be removed by inserting such filters in the light path of the microscope.

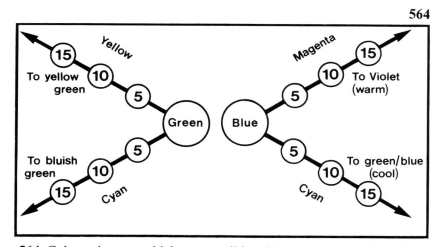

564

**564** Colour changes which are possible with weak 'fine tuning' filters.

## A  Film speed test

Most colour films are designed to satisfy the demands of a mass market and it is assumed that exposure times, subject contrast and other factors approximate to studio or daylight conditions. When these films are subjected to the extreme conditions imposed by photomicrography, such assumptions are not always valid. An initial working film speed test, therefore, is usually necessary.

On most modern cameras, film speed tests can be carried out rapidly by changing the ASA/Din film speed setting to give a bracketed series of exposures (each setting = ⅓ stop) over a total range of ± 2 stops at each side of the recommended rating. This should result in a series of transparencies ranging from under to over exposure from which it is easy to select the optimum practical film speed when viewed on a light box. Microscopes fitted with compur shutters or electronic flash equipment will require an appropriately modified technique to achieve the same end result.

Traditionally, photomicroscopists have used several different bracketing ratios as well as the standard 2×F numbers series. The more gradual 1.4 × sequence is often advocated, as are the Fibonacci series and approximations to it such as the 1.6 × ratio.

**565-568** *Bone marrow cells from a healthy grey heron, photographed on a Kodachrome II (professional, daylight) film with 80C and didymium filters at different ASA settings.*

**565**
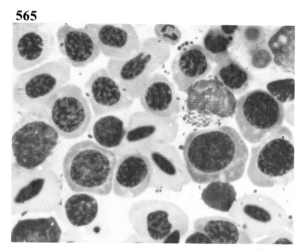
ASA 12

**566**
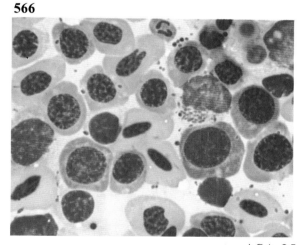
ASA 25

**567**
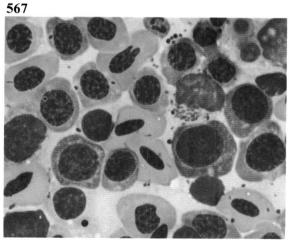
ASA 50

**568**
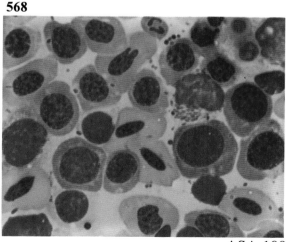
ASA 100

## B Exposure latitude test

For critical application, further tests within the limits of the normal 'correct exposure' range are helpful. These can be used to establish 'film speeds' for correct emphasis of either highlight detail, midtones or shadows.

For this, a range of ASA settings between those which appear within the acceptable exposure range in test **A** are used. This is usually one stop either side of the optimum exposure.

**569-572** *The same field photographed with the same film and filters as* **A** *but using a narrower range of ASA settings between ASA 25 and 64.*

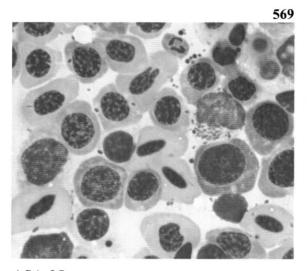

569

ASA 25

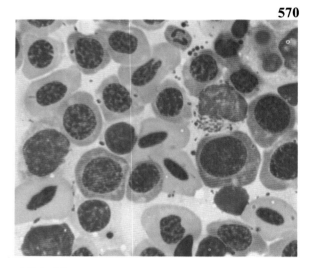

570

ASA 32

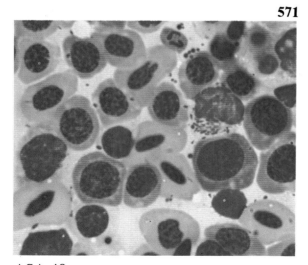

571

ASA 40

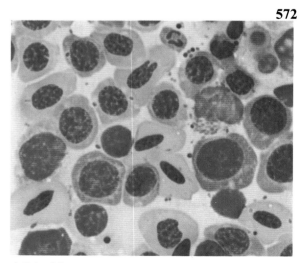

572

ASA 64

## C Colour temperature correction test

For optimum results, the colour of the illuminating source must match that of the film. A colour temperature difference of even a few degrees will result in transparencies showing a colour cast of blue if the temperature is too high or yellow/orange if it is too low. This blue/orange balance can be controlled by inserting appropriate colour temperature correcting filters in the light source. Suitable quality sets of filters in optical plastic are commercially available at low cost (Cokin filters) or in the form of sheets which can be cut to size (Lee filters).

**573-576** *The same field and film as* **A**, *using a graded series of colour temperature correction filters.*

**573**

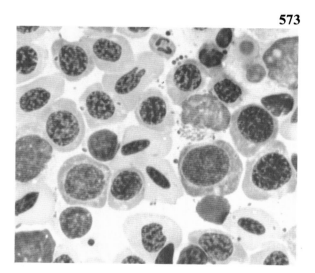

No filter

**574**

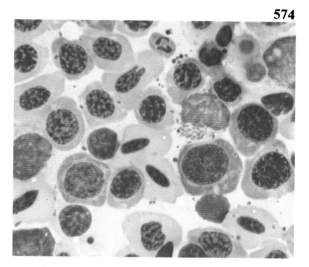

Lee ¼ CT blue

**575**

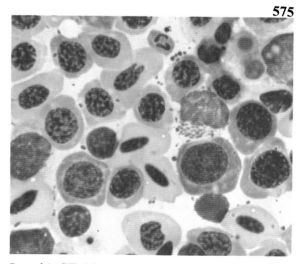

Lee ½ CT blue

**576**

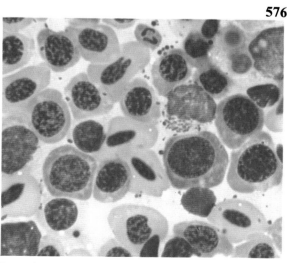

Lee full CT blue

## D Fine tuning test

A number of factors apart from the quality of the illumination can influence the colours in a transparency. Among the most common are film ageing, manufacturing variations and reciprocity failure (Table **4**). Compensation for these factors is achieved by using additional selective filtration with weak filters such as the compensating filters supplied for colour printing. To avoid overcorrection and the production of a complementary colour cast requiring further filtration, density values should not normally exceed CC 10 to CC 15.

## Table 4   Typical faults in colour reproduction

| Colour of subject | Typical fault | Colour of subject | Typical fault |
|---|---|---|---|
| RED | Orange shift<br>May reproduce too light | YELLOW | Often desaturated |
| ORANGE | May reproduce too light | GREEN & CYAN | Blue shift |
| PINK | Bluish shift | MAGNENTA | Red Shift |
| | | PURPLE | Red Shift |

**577-579** *Blood cells photographed on Kodachrome II (professional daylight) ASA 25 film with different colour correction filters.*

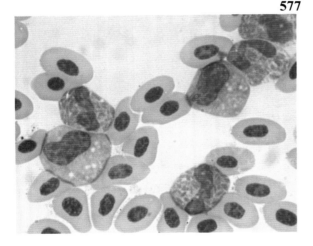

577

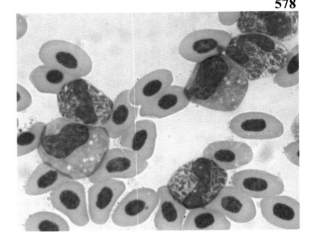

578

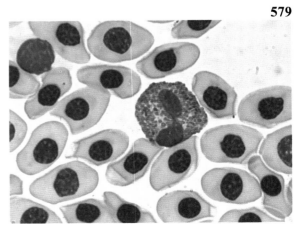

579

**577** Filters 80C + 10C, emphasising the monocytes. (Blood cells from a domestic fowl with *Mycobacterium avium* infection.)

**578** Filters 80C + 10B, emphasising the cytoplasmic granules of the heterophils. (Same field as **577**.)

**579** Filters 80C + 10Y, emphasising the colour of the red cell cytoplasm and the heterophil granules. (Blood cells from a plated lizard.)

## E  Colour speed/optimum saturation test

Significant variation in brightness of many colours in the transparency can be produced by the judicious use of under or over exposure. The effect will be consistent with a given range of colours on a particular make of film. The average (midtone) exposure tends to favour the flesh tones and landscape colours red, orange and blue-green. Lighter colours achieve their best saturation levels with a slightly less than average exposure time and darker colours such as blue, red and violet are improved by increased exposure (Table 5). Any changes made must be within the limits of the latitude of the film concerned and with regard to other colours in the subject which will be proportionally lightened or darkened according to their spectral position. With this system an important cell colour can be emphasised simply by changing the film speed setting to match the 'colour speed index' for that particular colour.

# Table 5  Typical colour speed/optimum saturation test

| Colour | ASA film speed | Relative neutral density change | F stop equivalent |
|---|---|---|---|
| YELLOW | 50 | + 0.3 | −1 stop |
| YELLOW-ORANGE/ YELLOW-GREEN | 40 | + 0.2 | −2⁄3 stop |
| ORANGE/GREEN | 32 | + 0.1 | − 1⁄3 stop |
| RED-ORANGE/GREEN-BLUE | 25 | none | rated speed |
| RED/BLUE | 20 | − 0.1 | + 1⁄3 stop |
| RED-VIOLET/BLUE-VIOLET | 16 | − 0.2 | + 2⁄3 stop |
| VIOLET | 12 | − 0.3 | + 1 stop |

Bracketed tests undertaken earlier provide the basis for a 'colour speed index'. For this test, a microscope slide which has a field containing examples of all the types of stained cells normally encountered should be selected. Alternatively, a colour chart can be photographed under conditions which approximate to those used in photomicrography, as shown in **580-587**.

**580-587** *Colour chart photographed on Ektachrome 100 (professional, daylight) film.*

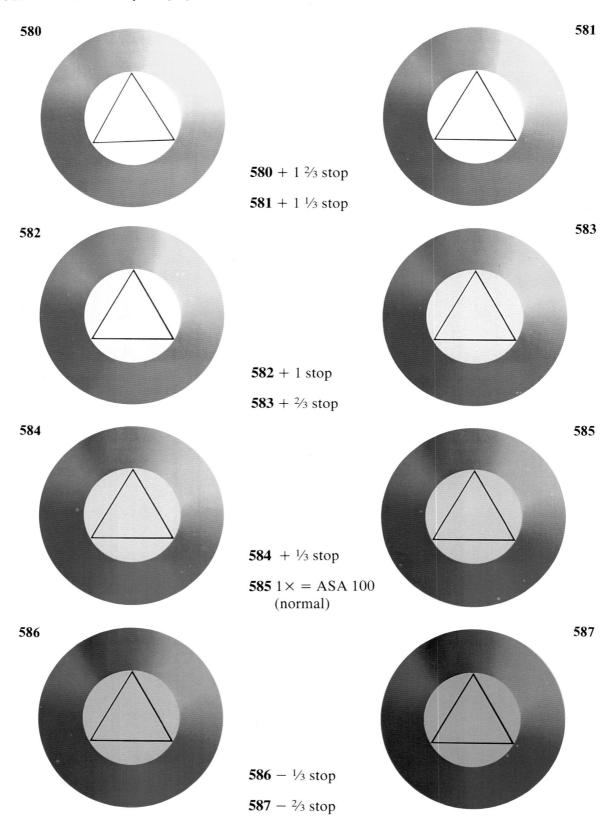

**580**

**581**

**580** + 1 ⅔ stop

**581** + 1 ⅓ stop

**582**

**583**

**582** + 1 stop

**583** + ⅔ stop

**584**

**585**

**584** + ⅓ stop

**585** 1× = ASA 100
(normal)

**586**

**587**

**586** − ⅓ stop

**587** − ⅔ stop

## F Film selection test

The products of different manufacturers vary considerably in colour, sensitivity and overall tonality. North American (Kodak) Standard Films have a warm bias whereas European (D.I.N) Standard (Agfa) are cool. Current Japanese films (Fuji, Konica) and the new generation of Kodak 'professional films' show enhanced sensitivity to particular colours, to give improved reproduction of bright Azo fabric dyes encountered by the fashion photographer. These differences constitute a valuable tool for the photomicroscopist since, by using films of different manufacturers, it is possible to overcome several commonly encountered problems.

**588-591** *Blood cells from a plated lizard photographed on different films.*

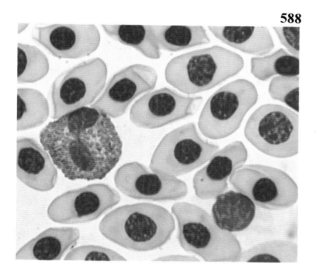

**588**

Kodachrome II (professional, daylight) film, ASA 25, filter 80B

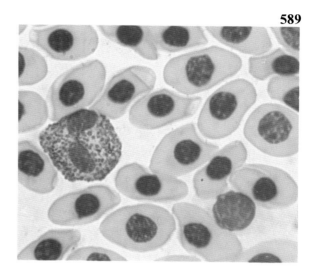

**589**

Agfachrome 50 RS, filter 80B

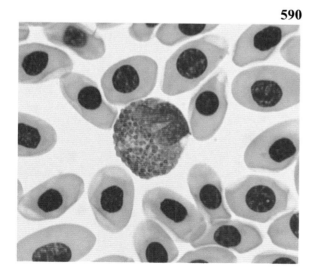

**590**

Fuji 50, filter 80B

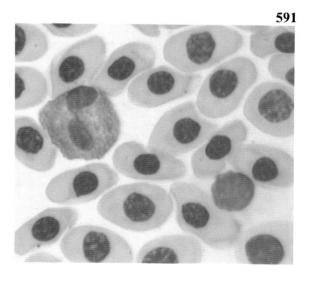

**591**

Ektachrome 100, filter 10B

## G Colour correction

A number of dyes, including eosin and fuchin, do not reproduce well on modern colour films and many histological dyes are of a higher saturation than used in current photographic emulsions. Additionally, some films are sensitive to ultraviolet light which, although invisible to the eye, will record as excess blue on film. Compensation for these factors can be made by selective filtration, either by adjusting the colour temperature correction filters with an additional filter pack, or by constructing a single basic filter pack from colour compensating filters to take all factors into consideration. Kodachrome films, however, require a very narrow cut filter to overcome the reduced spectral response to light reddish stains. The didymium filter referred to previously provides a simple means of controlling this problem.

**592-593** *Bone marrow cells from a grey heron photographed on Kodachrome II (professional, daylight) film with and without a didymium filter.*

**592**

**593**

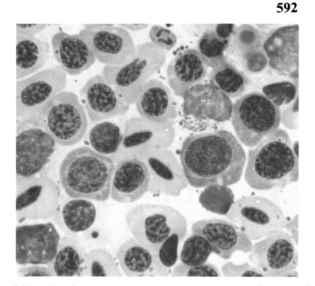
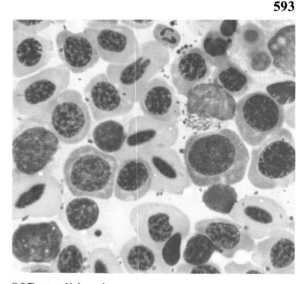

80B (basic colour temperature correction) only   80B + didymium

In applying corrective filters, it is sometimes found that the optimum cell colour can be achieved only at the expense of background neutrality. While a white or neutral background may be desirable photographically, it is of little importance diagnostically, when the correct rendering of variation in specimen colour is the ultimate goal.

**594-601** *Blood cells from an anaconda photographed with different filter combinations.*

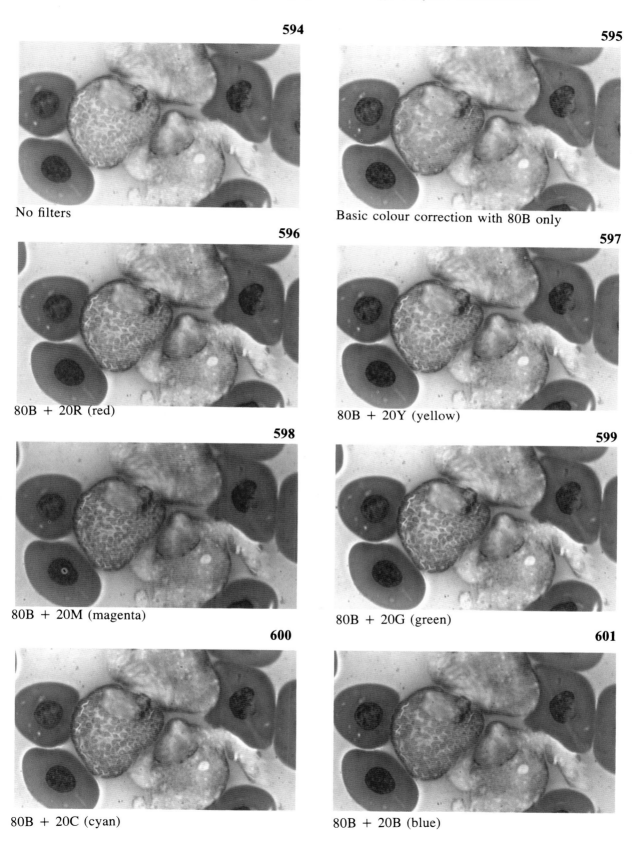

**594**

No filters

**595**

Basic colour correction with 80B only

**596**

80B + 20R (red)

**597**

80B + 20Y (yellow)

**598**

80B + 20M (magenta)

**599**

80B + 20G (green)

**600**

80B + 20C (cyan)

**601**

80B + 20B (blue)

# Species list

## MAMMALS

| | | |
|---|---|---|
| MONOTREMATA | Bruijn's echidna | *Zaglossus bruijni* |
| MARSUPIALIA | Red-necked wallaby | *Macropus rufogriseus* |
| SCANDENTIA | Large tree shrew | *Tupaia tana* |
| CHIROPTERA | Fruit bat | *Epomophorus gambianus parvus* |
| PRIMATES | Brown lemur | *Lemur fulvus* |
| | Ruffed lemur | *Varecia variegatus* |
| | Grey mouse lemur | *Microcebus murinus* |
| | Slender loris | *Loris tardigradus* |
| | Owl monkey (=Douroucouli) | *Aotus trivirgatus* |
| | White-headed Saki | *Pithecia pithecia* |
| | Brown capuchin | *Cebus apella* |
| | Squirrel monkey | *Samiri sciureus* |
| | Black spider monkey | *Ateles paniscus* |
| | Long-haired spider monkey | *Ateles belzebuth* |
| | Common marmoset | *Callithrix jacchus* |
| | Silvery marmoset | *Callithrix argentata* |
| | Cotton-top tamarin | *Saguinus oedipus* |
| | Red-bellied tamarin | *Saguinus labiatus* |
| | Rhesus macaque | *Macaca mulatta* |
| | Crab-eating (=Cynomolgus) macaque | *Macaca fascicularis* |
| | Lion-tailed macaque | *Macaca silenus* |
| | Barbary ape | *Macaca sylvanus* |
| | Anubis baboon | *Papio anubis* |
| | Vervet monkey | *Cercopithecus aethiops* |
| | Orang utan | *Pongo pygmaeus* |
| | Chimpanzee | *Pan troglodytes* |
| | Man | *Homo sapiens* |
| EDENTATA | Giant anteater | *Myrmecophaga tridactyla* |
| | Two-toed sloth | *Choloepus didactylus* |
| LAGOMORPHA | European (=Domestic) rabbit | *Oryctolagus cuniculus* |
| RODENTIA | Grey squirrel | *Sciurus carolinensis* |
| | Prairie marmot | *Cynomys ludovicianus* |
| | Canadian beaver | *Castor canadensis* |
| | European (=common) hamster | *Cricetus cricetus* |
| | Giant rat | *Cricetomys gambianus* |
| | Brown (=Laboratory) rat | *Rattus norvegicus* |
| | House (=Laboratory) mouse | *Mus musculus* |
| | Guinea pig | *Cavia porcellus* |
| | Mara | *Dolichotis patagonum* |
| | Capybara | *Hydrochoerus hydrochaeris* |
| | Plains viscacha | *Lagostomus maximus* |
| | Jamaican hutia | *Geocapromys brownii* |
| | Casiragua | *Proechimys guariae* |

| CARNIVORA | Grey wolf | *Canis lupus* |
| | Domestic dog | *Canis familiaris* |
| | Polar bear | *Thalarctos maritimus* |
| | Polecat (=Domestic ferret) | *Mustela putorius* |
| | Ring-tailed coati | *Nasua nasua* |
| | Hog badger | *Arctonyx collaris* |
| | Blotched genet | *Genetta tigrina* |
| | Masked palm civet | *Paguma larvata* |
| | Indian brown mongoose | *Herpestes edwardsi* |
| | Crab-eating mongoose | *Herpestes urva* |
| | Domestic cat | *Felis catus* |
| | Lion | *Panthera leo* |
| | Tiger | *Panthera tigris* |
| | Leopard | *Panthera pardus* |
| | Jaguar | *Panthera onca* |
| | Cheetah | *Acinonyx jubatus* |
| | | |
| PINNIPEDIA | Californian sealion | *Zalophus californianus* |
| | | |
| CETACEA | Bottle-nosed dolphin | *Tursiops truncatus* |
| | | |
| PROBOSCIDEA | Indian elephant | *Elephas maximus* |
| | | |
| PERISSODACTYLA | Domestic horse | *Equus caballus* |
| | Donkey (=African wild ass) | *Equus asinus* |
| | Wild horse | *Equus przewalskii* |
| | White rhinoceros | *Ceratotherium simum* |
| | | |
| ARTIODACTYLA | Wild boar (=Domestic pig) | *Sus scrofa* |
| | Collared peccary | *Tayassu tajacu* |
| | Hippopotamus | *Hippopotamus amphibius* |
| | Llama | *Lama glama* |
| | Alpaca | *Lama pacos* |
| | Bactrian camel | *Camelus bactrianus* |
| | Arabian camel (=Dromedary) | *Camelus dromedarius* |
| | Reeves' muntjac | *Muntiacus reevesi* |
| | Fallow deer | *Dama dama* |
| | Red deer | *Cervus elaphus* |
| | Swamp deer (=Barasingha) | *Cervus duvauceli* |
| | Père David's deer | *Elaphurus davidianus* |
| | Reindeer | *Rangifer tarandus* |
| | Moose | *Alces alces* |
| | Eland | *Taurotragus oryx* |
| | Nilgai | *Boselaphus tragocamelus* |
| | Gaur | *Bos gaurus* |
| | Domestic ox (=Cattle) | *Bos taurus* |
| | Yak | *Bos grunniens* |
| | African buffalo | *Syncerus caffer* |
| | Asiatic (=Domestic) buffalo | *Bubalus bubalus* |
| | European bison | *Bison bonasus* |
| | Roan antelope | *Hippotragus equinus* |
| | Scimitar-horned oryx | *Oryx tao* |
| | Arabian oryx | *Oryx leucoryx* |
| | Blesbok | *Damaliscus dorcas* |
| | Domestic goat | *Capra hircus* |
| | Markhor | *Capra falconeri* |
| | Domestic sheep | *Ovis aries* |
| | Bighorn sheep | *Ovis canadensis* |

# BIRDS

| | | |
|---|---|---|
| STRUTHIONIFORMES | Ostrich | *Struthio camelus* |
| CASUARIIFORMES | Emu | *Dromaius novaehollandiae* |
| SPHENISCIFORMES | Black-footed penguin | *Spheniscus demersus* |
| CICONIIFORMES | Marabou stork | *Leptoptilos crumeniferus* |
| | White stork | *Ciconia ciconia* |
| | Sacred ibis | *Threskiornis aethiopicus* |
| | Roseate spoonbill | *Platalea leucorodia* |
| | Rosy flamingo | *Phoenicopterus ruber ruber* |
| | Grey heron | *Ardea cinerea* |
| FALCONIFORMES | Common buzzard | *Buteo buteo* |
| | Golden eagle | *Aquila chrysaetos* |
| | Sparrowhawk | *Accipiter nisus* |
| | Goshawk | *Accipiter gentilis* |
| | Lappet-faced vulture | *Torgos tracheliotus* |
| GALLIFORMES | Domestic fowl | *Gallus gallus* |
| | North American (=Domestic) turkey | *Meleagris gallipavo* |
| | Mikado pheasant | *Syrmaticus mikado* |
| | Yellow-necked spurfowl | *Francolinus leucoscepus* |
| ANSERIFORMES | Whooper swan | *Cygnus cygnus cygnus* |
| | Mallard (=Domestic duck) | *Anas platyrhynchos* |
| | Domestic goose | *Anser* spp. |
| GRUIFORMES | Sarus crane | *Grus antigone* |
| | Hooded crane | *Grus monacha* |
| | Crowned crane | *Balearica pavonina gibbericeps* |
| | Moorhen | *Gallinula chloropus* |
| | Kori bustard | *Choriotis kori* |
| COLUMBIFORMES | Rock dove (=Domestic pigeon) | *Columba livia* |
| | Cape turtle dove | *Streptopelia capicola* |
| PSITTACIFORMES | Yellow-backed lory | *Lorius garrulus flavopalliatus* |
| | Lesser sulphur-crested cockatoo | *Cacatua sulphurea* |
| | Moluccan cockatoo | *Cacatua moluccensis* |
| | Budgerigar | *Melopsittacus undulatus* |
| | Grey parrot | *Psittacus erithacus* |
| | Yellow-fronted Amazon parrot | *Amazona ochrocephala* |
| | Blue and gold macaw | *Ara ararauna* |
| | Buffon's macaw | *Ara ambigua* |
| STRIGIFORMES | Javan fish owl | *Ketupa ketupa* |
| | Snowy owl | *Nyctea scandiaca* |
| | Tawny owl | *Strix aluco* |
| | Little owl | *Athene noctua* |
| CORACIIFORMES | Kookaburra | *Dacelo novaeguineae* |
| PROCELLARIIFORMES | Wandering albatross | *Diomedea exulans* |

184

| PASSERIFORMES | Blue tit | *Parus caeruleus* |
| | Blue waxbill | *Uraeginthus angolensis* |
| | Canary | *Serinus canaria* |
| | Dark plain-backed pipit | *Anthus leucophrys* |
| | Hill mynah | *Gracula religiosa* |
| | House sparrow | *Passer domesticus* |
| | Olive thrush | *Turdus abyssinicus* |
| | Puffback shrike | *Dryoscopus cubla* |
| | Red-billed blue magpie | *Urocissa erythrorhyncha* |
| | Scarlet-chested sunbird | *Nectarinia senegalensis* |
| | Wattled starling | *Creatophora cinerea* |
| | White-eared bulbul | *Pycnonotus barbatus dodsoni* |

# REPTILES

| TESTUDINES | Hawksbill turtle | *Eretmochelys imbricata* |
| | Peacock soft-shelled turtle | *Trionyx hurum* |
| | Red-eared terrapin | *Chrysemys scripta elegans* |
| | Spur-thighed tortoise | *Testudo graeca* |
| | Hermann's tortoise | *Testudo hermanni* |
| | Aldabra giant tortoise | *Geochelone gigantea* |
| | Yellow-footed tortoise | *Geochelone dendiculata* |

| CROCODYLIA | Nile crocodile | *Crocodylus niloticus* |
| | Mississippi alligator | *Alligator mississippiensis* |
| | Chinese alligator | *Alligator sinensis* |

| SAURIA | Common iguana | *Iguana iguana* |
| | Rhinoceros iguana | *Cyclura cornutus* |
| | Shingleback skink | *Trachydosaurus rugosus* |
| | Blue-tongued skink | *Tiliqua scincoides scincoides* |
| | Greater plated lizard | *Gerrhosaurus major* |
| | Gila monster | *Heloderma suspectum* |
| | Nile monitor | *Varanus niloticus* |
| | Green waterdragon | *Physignathus cocincinus* |
| | LeSueur's water dragon | *Physignathus lesueurii* |
| | Black-pointed tegu | *Tupinanbis nigropunctatus* |
| | Green lizard | *Lacerta viridis* |

| SERPENTES | Rock python | *Python molurus bivittatus* |
| | Indian python | *Python molurus molurus* |
| | Royal python | *Python regius* |
| | Reticulated python | *Python reticulatus* |
| | African python | *Python sebae* |
| | Carpet python | *Morelia spilotis* |
| | Brown python | *Liasis fuscus* |
| | Rat snake | *Elaphe obsoleta* |
| | Fox snake | *Elaphe vulpina* |
| | Taipan snake | *Oxyuranus scutellatus* |
| | Gaboon viper | *Bitis gabonica* |
| | Boomslang | *Dispholidus typus* |
| | Boa constrictor | *Boa constrictor* |
| | Black mamba | *Dendroaspis polylepis* |
| | Montpelier snake | *Malpolon monspessulanus* |
| | Anaconda | *Eunectes notaeus* |
| | Mozambique spitting cobra | *Naja mossambica* |
| | Seychelles house snake | *Boaedon geometricus* |
| | Zambian house snake | *Boaedon fuliginosus* |

# GLOSSARY

| | |
|---|---|
| ANISOCYTOSIS | Variation in cell size. |
| BASOPHILIC STIPPLING | Describes the presence of a variable number of basophilic granules in red cells. |
| CRENATION | The process by which red cells develop many projections at their surface. Usually considered to be a technical artefact. |
| DOHLE (AMATO) BODIES | Small blue-staining areas in the cytoplasm of neutrophils and eosinophils, probably representing localised failure of maturation. |
| ECHINOCYTES (*BURR CELLS*) | Red cells with one or more spiney projections. |
| ELLIPTOCYTES | Oval red cells. |
| HEINZ BODIES | Intra-erythrocytic inclusions representing denatured (non-functional) haemoglobin. Can vary in size, shape and number. Visible in cells stained supravitally with new methylene blue but not with Romanowsky stains. |
| HOWELL JOLLY BODIES | Excentric, round purple red cell inclusions containing DNA and representing nuclear remnants. |
| HYPOCHROMIA | Reduced haemoglobin content. |
| LEFT SHIFT | Decreased nuclear lobulation. |
| MACROCYTOSIS | Increased cell size. |
| MICROCYTOSIS | Decreased cell size. |
| PELGER-HUET PHENOMENON | Harmless inherited condition where neutrophils (and possibly other granulocytic cells) show decreased nuclear lobulation. Described in man, dogs, cats, rabbits, bactrian camels and white rhinoceroses. |
| POIKILOCYTOSIS | Irregular shape. |
| POLYCHROMASIA (*POLYCHROMIA*) | Red cells staining with a basophilic tinge, indicating incomplete haemoglobin formation. |
| RETICULOCYTES | Newly released red cells containing reticular material which stains supravitally with new methylene blue stain but not with Romanowsky stains. |
| RIGHT SHIFT | Increased number of nuclear lobes. |
| ROULEAUX | The face-to-face contact of discocytic red cells to form stacks of various lengths and conformations. |
| SCHISTOCYTES | Red cell fragments. |
| SICKLE CELLS (*DREPANOCYTES*) | Red cells which show a reversible shape change involving the development of two (or more) projections. |
| SPHEROCYTES | Red cells which are thicker than normal. |
| STOMATOCYTES | Red cells with a slit-like central area of pallor or appearing cup-shaped in thick parts of a blood film. |
| TARGET (*MEXICAN HAT*) CELLS | Red cells with a central red-staining area surrounded by an unstained or paler staining ring. |
| TOXIC GRANULATION | Abnormal basophilic granules in the cytoplasm of neutrophils (and heterophils?), indicating disturbed granule formation resulting in decreased intracellular lysosome content. |

# BIBLIOGRAPHY

Allen, R.M. 1958. *Photomicography*. D. Van Nostrand, New York.

Andrew, W. 1965. *Comparative Hematology*. Grune & Stratton, New York and London.

Archer, R.K. & Jeffcott, L.B.(Eds.) 1977. *Comparative Clinical Haematology*. Blackwell, Oxford.

Dein, F.J. 1984. *Laboratory Manual of Avian Hematology*. Association of Avian Veterinarians, East Northport, N.Y.

Frye, F.L. 1981. *Biomedical and Surgical aspects of captive Reptile Husbandry*. Veterinary Medicine Publishing Co., Edwardsville, Kansas.

Garnham, P.C.C. 1966. *Malarial Parasites and other Haemosporidia*. Blackwell, Oxford.

Hawkey, C.M. 1975. *Comparative Mammalian Haematology* . Heinemann Medical Books, London.

Hayhoe, H.J. & Flemens, R.J. 1982. *A Colour Atlas of Haematological Cytology*. Wolfe Medical Publications, London.

Hoar, C.A. 1972. *The Trypanosomes of Mammals*. Blackwell, Oxford.

Huser, H.J. 1970. *Atlas of Comparative Primate Hematology*. Academic Press, New York & London.

Jain, N.C. 1986. *Schalm's Veterinary Haematology*. Lea & Febiger, Philadelphia.

Keller, P. & Freudiger, U. 1984. *Atlas of Hematology of the Dog and Cat*. Paul Parey, Hamburg.

Klosevych, S. 1964. Photomicography – resolution and magnification. *J. Biol. Phot. Assoc*. 32:4.

Lawson, D.F. 1960. *The Technique of Photomicography*. MacMillan Co., New York.

Loveland, R.P. 1970. *Photomicography, a comprehensive treatise*. John Wiley & Sons Inc., New York.

Lucas, A.M. & Jamroz, C. 1961. *Atlas of Avian Hematology*. Agriculture Monograph 25, United States Department of Agriculture, Washington D.C.

Needham, G.H. 1958. *The Practical Use of the Microscope*. Charles C. Thomas, Springfield, Illinois.

Ohta, N. 1984. *The color gamut obtainable by combination of subtractive color dyes*. Scientific Publications of the Fuji Photo Film Co. Ltd., no 29.

Pienaar, U. de V. 1962. *Haematology of some South African Reptiles*. Witwatersrand University Press, Johannesburg.

Sanderson J.H. & Phillips, C.E. 1981. *An Atlas of Laboratory Animal Haematology*. Clarendon Press, Oxford.

Schalm, O.W., Jain, N.C. & Carroll, E.J. 1975. *Veterinary Hematology*. Lea & Febiger, Philadelphia.

Schermer, S. 1967. *The Blood Morphology of Laboratory Animals*. (3rd. ed.), F.A. Davis Company, Philadelphia.

Schreiber, D. 1960. *Introduction to the morphology of blood*. Veb Georg Thieme, Leipzig.

Spinell, B.M. 1961. Simplified 35mm photomicography with improved results. *J. Biol. Phot. Assoc*. 29:4.

# Species Index

Figures in **bold** type denote illustrations; those in light type denote pages.

# Subject Index

Figures in **bold** type denote illustrations; those in light type denote pages.